Vital Nephrology

Your *essential* reference for
all aspects of renal care

Andy Stein MD, MRCP
Consultant Nephrologist and General Physician,
University Hospitals, Coventry and Warwickshire NHS Trust

Janet Wild RGN
Clinical Education Manager,
Baxter Healthcare Ltd,
Newbury, Berkshire

Paul Cook MSc, MRCP
Renal Registrar,
Hammersmith Hospital

Class Health • London

Printing history
First published 2004

The authors and publishers welcome feedback from the users of this book. Please contact the publishers.
Class Publishing, Barb House, Barb Mews, London W6 7PA, UK
Telephone: 020 7371 2119
Fax: 020 7371 2878 [International +4420]
email: post@class.co.uk
Visit our website – www.class.co.uk

A CIP catalogue for this book is available from the British Library

ISBN 1 85959 102 7

Edited and indexed by Richenda Milton-Thompson

Designed and typeset by Martin Bristow

Line illustrations by David Woodroffe

Printed and bound in Slovenia by Delo Tiskarna by arrangement with Presernova druzba

Contents

Introduction

It wasn't until quite late in life that I discovered how to say, "I don't know" – W Somerset Maugham

Nephrology is a vast subject. It would be impossible for us to summarise it all in one short book. However, we hope we have written a useful 'fact file' of information about the most vital points of nephrology. It is not meant to be a tome. It is a 'practical book', helping the reader with day-to-day decisions – for example, how to set up a renal biopsy, but not how to interpret it. Other books can tell you that.

It has been written for all renal unit health professionals. But it is especially aimed at ward doctors and nurses. Even so, we hope it will be useful to house officers, and more junior nurses – and indeed to specialist registrars and consultants who are looking for practical, easily accessible information. We have tried to concentrate on the issues that arise most frequently in the ward situation and steer away from the outpatients' domain, admittedly where most renal patients are seen.

We hope it will give you the right type of information, in situations where there is no one around to ask, or when you feel you should already know the answer. The standards set by the Renal Association – to which we should all aspire – are integral to the text.

Each chapter includes a 'patient education' section. This is designed partly to help the health professional with words to describe complicated or delicate topics to patients; and partly for the occasional patient-reader.

We (Andy Stein and Janet Wild) recruited the help of Dr Paul Cook, a Specialist Renal Registrar, as we felt we were now too far from the coalface to write about what actually happens there. Without his help, this book would not have been written. He fitted in seamlessly to an established writing team.

Finally, the book could not have been readable without our 'own editor' (this is the third book she has helped us with) – Richenda Milton-Thompson. We would like to thank Peter McGarry, a patient of Andy's, for the inspiration to write about 'non-concordance'; though we would like to point out that he himself is entirely in concord with all medical requests of course! In addition we would like to thank our reviewers Professor Terry Feest, Dr Kelly Hunt, Dr Phin Kon, Althea Mahon, Dr Steve Nelson and Dr Daniel Zehnder. Dr Vicki Ayub provided invaluable help with the chapters on dialysis, Juliet Auer with the sections on discontinuing dialysis and bereavement, and Hayley Jones with the appendix on prescribing. And of course, this list would not be complete without mention of Richard (Dick) Warner of Class Publishing, who has encouraged us every step of the way.

Inevitably, different units have different protocols, so we have tried to write for the majority. If anything differs wildly from what you do in your unit, or you think we have got anything wrong, please let us know.

Andy Stein, Janet Wild and Paul Cook
Coventry, Manchester and London

1 Chronic renal failure (CRF)

The whole of this chapter, and most of this book, is about chronic renal failure (CRF) and its treatment.

Functions

The kidneys have four main functions:

- Excretory - excretion of waste products and drugs
- Regulatory - regulation of water and electrolyte balance (and hence blood pressure)
- Endocrine - production of erythropoietin, renin and prostaglandins
- Metabolic - metabolism of vitamin D

As a consequence CRF can cause fluid overload, hypertension, anaemia and bone disease.

Definitions

- Chronic renal failure is a permanent, usually progressive, reduction in renal function
- End-stage renal failure (ESRF) is an advanced stage of CRF that results in death unless some form of renal replacement therapy is initiated

Epidemiology

(Data taken from UK Renal Registry, 2003)

- The current median age of presentation in the UK is 64 years
- It is more common in men (63.2% of new patients are male)
- Compared to a white population, the incidence of ESRF is 3-5 times greater in Asian and Black populations in the UK

The size of the problem

- Renal failure is a relatively minor public health problem when compared to ischaemic heart disease, diabetes and cancer. But the expense of renal replacement therapy means it uses a disproportionate amount of health care resources
- The incidence of ESRF in adults in the UK in 2001 was 93.2 per million population (pmp) for adults
- The prevalence of ESRF in the UK on 31 December 2001 was 566 pmp. This equates to 33,363 people
- By the start of the 21st century nearly one million people worldwide were being treated by dialysis for ESRF

Diagnosis and progression

Many patients have a silent illness of insidious onset, with few symptoms. So it is often an unexpected (biochemical) diagnosis, made by blood tests carried out for other reasons.

- **Renal failure** is usually diagnosed by measuring the serum creatinine. However, measurement of the glomerular filtration rate (GFR) is necessary to define the exact level of renal function. It is important to appreciate that the serum urea and creatinine may not rise above the normal range until GFR is reduced by 50%. An accurate measurement of GFR can be achieved by performing an isotopic GFR using EDTA

- **Creatinine clearance** is often used as an estimate of GFR (a normal GFR is 80-120 ml/min). It is most useful when there is normal or near normal renal function and can be conveniently measured using the Cockcroft-Gault equation:

In men:
$$\text{Creatinine clearance} = \frac{(140 - \text{age}) \times \text{weight in kg}}{(72 \times \text{serum creatinine } \mu\text{mol/l})}$$

In women:
$$\text{Creatinine clearance} = \frac{(140 - \text{age}) \times \text{weight in kg}}{(72 \times \text{serum creatinine } \mu\text{mol/l})} \times 0.85$$

** A normal serum urea or creatinine
is not synonymous with a normal GFR*

CRF usually progresses to ESRF. This occurs over a period of months, years or even decades. It cannot usually be cured, but there are interventions that can slow progression and improve symptoms. ESRF is best dealt with by a multiprofessional team of nephrologist, nurse, dietitian, social worker, counsellor, transplant co-ordinator and transplant surgeon. There is no doubt that early planning for renal replacement therapy improves outcomes.

Causes of ESRF

There are many causes of chronic renal failure. Listed below are those that commonly account for ESRF in the UK (Renal Registry, 2003):

- Diabetes (18.6%)
- Glomerulonephritis (12.5%)
- Reflux nephropathy (10.2%)
- Renovascular (6.9%)
- Hypertension (6.8%)
- Autosomal dominant polycystic kidney disease (6.7%)

** Diabetes mellitus is now the most common identifiable
cause of ESRF, being present in nearly 20% of new patients*

Renal presentation syndromes

There are only **eight** renal presentation syndromes:
1. Asymptomatic proteinuria
2. Nephrotic syndrome
3. Microscopic haematuria
4. Macroscopic haematuria
5. Nephritic syndrome
6. Hypertension
7. Acute renal failure
8. Chronic renal failure

Clinical features of CRF

- CRF can affect every organ system. Uraemia is a clinical state of poisoning by products of endogenous catabolism. The most serious manifestation of CRF is the uraemic emergency. This is characterised by:
  - Pulmonary oedema
  - Hyperkalaemia
  - Metabolic acidosis
  - Uraemic/hypertensive encephalopathy
  - Pericarditis/pericardial tamponade
- Beware shortness of breath in a patient with CRF. Although it is often multifactorial (fluid overload, anaemia and acidosis), fluid overload is by far the most important contributing cause
- Low potassium can cause paralysis of the leg muscles. But high potassium can give rise to the same symptom

VITAL POINT

* A patient who says their legs don't work properly may have life-threatening hyperkalaemia ... test potassium levels immediately!

(Management of hyperkalaemia is similar to that of acute renal failure - see pages 34-39)

Treatment options

The optimal choice of renal replacement therapy will be different for different patients at varying stages of their illness. There are three modes of renal replacement therapy:

■ Haemodialysis/haemofiltration

■ Peritoneal dialysis

■ Renal transplantation

When do you start treatment?

■ There is no simple answer to this question. Studies (usually retrospective) of early versus late dialysis show no obvious gain in life expectancy as a result of starting treatment early. Advantages in terms of quality of life are another matter, however

■ Dialysis (or a predialysis transplant) should be considered when the GFR is 10-15 ml/min, depending on symptoms. This may equate to a creatinine of 400-800 µmol/l, depending on age, sex and muscle mass

■ An early start of dialysis (or a transplant) in patients with predictably steadily progressive renal failure (eg autosomal dominant polycystic kidney disease - ADPKD - or glomerulonephritis) is practical. Those with relatively stable renal function, however, may often be treated conservatively for longer

Slowing progression

The rate of decline of renal function varies between patients and between diseases. However, irrespective of the initial disease, common mechanisms underlie progression at a pathophysiological level. The key clinical risk factors that make progression more likely are:

■ Proteinuria - the higher the level the more rapid the decline

■ Hypertension

Therefore the most important therapeutic interventions are:

- Blood pressure control targets are 125/75 mmHg for those with progressive proteinuric renal disease and 130/80 for those with stable renal function. It probably does not matter that much *how* you get the BP down, just get it down

- Angiotensin converting enzyme (ACE) inhibitors (or AII blockers) should be considered as the agents of first choice in patients with progressive proteinuric renal disease, whether hypertensive or not

VITAL POINT

* Screening for (and treating) microalbuminuria (ie 30–300 mg/24h) is thought to improve renal prognosis in those with type I diabetes mellitus

VITAL POINT

* ACE inhibitors and AII blockers reduce proteinuria and delay the progression of proteinuric renal disease ('renoprotective') – and should be started early

Prognosis

- The mortality of the ESRF population is very high relative to the general population. It can be worse than for many types of cancer – the prognosis for ESRF is somewhere between colon and lung cancer

- In the UK, currently 79% of people are alive at the end of the first year of dialysis (90% of those under 45), and 48% at 4 years

- Cardiovascular disease is the most common cause of death

VITAL POINT

CRF cannot usually be cured. But it can be treated, often very effectively

Patient education

Tell them the vital point above, then tell them the others below – *slowly*:

- Your kidneys have four main functions:
  - ◆ To help you get rid of waste products and water
  - ◆ To regulate your blood pressure
  - ◆ To make essential substances including erythropoietin (EPO – used to make red blood cells)
  - ◆ To enable your body to make use of vitamin D (for strong bones)
- When your kidneys begin to fail, this is usually the start of an irreversible process – called chronic kidney (or 'renal') failure, CRF – that will often lead eventually to end-stage renal failure, ESRF
- Eventually, ESRF will need to be treated by dialysis or transplant, if you are to survive
- CRF can be diagnosed, and its progress monitored, by measuring the level of two substances, urea and creatinine, in your blood. The higher the blood levels, the worse your kidneys, dialysis or transplant are working
- Doctors do not always know why kidneys fail, but in many cases it is due to the effects of another disease such as diabetes mellitus
- Try to keep your blood pressure low if you have renal failure
- If you smoke, you really do need to give up. Take advantage of all the help available, from nicotine patches and gum, to hypnosis or counselling. See if your GP surgery runs a 'Stop Smoking' programme

Reference

Kimmel, P (2001) Management of the patient with chronic renal disease. In: Greenberg, A. (ed.) *Primer on kidney diseases*. Academic Press

2 Renal biopsy

- The decision to order a biopsy is NOT an SHO decision – it should be made by a consultant
- A renal biopsy can be performed on either a native kidney or a transplanted kidney
- It is an important tool in the diagnosis, management and prognosis of intrinsic renal disease
- However, it is a potentially dangerous procedure that can cause complications or even death
- The risks of renal biopsy should be compared with the benefits for each patient
- Would you have one in the same situation?

VITAL POINT

✶ Think about whether the biopsy is indicated and what it might show

Indications for renal biopsy

- You would assume that the consultant who has asked for a biopsy will know what he or she is doing
- Assume nothing
- Remember if it goes wrong (and the biopsy wasn't indicated) it's partly your fault
- The main indications for renal biopsy are:
  - ◆ Acute renal failure (ARF) with normal sized kidneys, and no obvious cause
  - ◆ Chronic renal failure (CRF) with normal sized kidneys, and no obvious cause

- Some patients with proteinuria (> 2g/24hr) and haematuria
- Renal transplant dysfunction

What's the best time?

- It is always best to do a kidney biopsy in the morning so that relevant emergency services are available should they be needed. If attempts are made to perform the biopsy out of hours or late in the day, ask why. If it's urgent, ring the pathologist. Ring the pathology technician. Take samples there yourself. Make sure everyone knows you want a 'same day' service
- If you work somewhere where they don't look at biopsies, get it to your local centre. Supervise its passage there yourself. Make sure a courier has been organised, and someone knows to tell you if it hasn't arrived by a certain time

Tests

Ensure these are done and the results recorded

- Full blood count, urea and electrolytes, clotting – within the last 24 hours; ask about bleeding tendency, eg at the dentist etc.
- Group and save
- Renal ultrasound . . . are there two kidneys? (Very important as you risk damaging one)
- Some units give desamino-D-arginine vasopressin (DDAVP) to improve platelet function in those with renal impairment (0.3 µg/kg IV one hour prior to the procedure)
- Stop aspirin and NSAIDs (7–10 days before the biopsy) and warfarin (4 days before the biopsy), and make sure no heparin is given on the day of biopsy or 24 hours afterwards

VITAL POINT

** For a native biopsy,
check the patient has two kidneys*

Patient education before the procedure

- A renal biopsy involves putting a large needle into you, and therefore requires your consent
- You will have a drip-needle inserted, but will not normally be sedated
- You will need to lie face down for biopsy of your own kidney, and on your back for biopsy of a transplanted kidney
- Your skin will be washed with antiseptic and local anaesthetic will be injected
- The doctor will use ultrasound to find the exact position of your kidney
- You will be asked to hold your breath (as this stops the kidney moving) and the biopsy is then performed (usually with a biopsy gun or Tru-cut needle). Two pieces ('cores') of tissue are obtained for native biopsies and one for transplant biopsies
- The whole process will take about one hour. You may be quite sore afterwards and will need to rest for about 12 hours

When NOT to do a biopsy

- Biopsies should be avoided if the patient has any of the following:
  - Systolic blood pressure > 160 mmHg; diastolic blood pressure > 95 mmHg
  - Haemoglobin < 8
  - Platelets < 100
  - INR or APTR > 1.2
  - Only one kidney (unless a transplant biopsy, or there is a very good reason to biopsy a single native kidney)
  - Obstructed kidneys
  - Small kidneys (< 10 cm)
- It is inadvisable to do a biopsy for the diagnosis of amyloid before other tissues have been biopsied (eg rectal biopsy) as they bleed

Complications

- The main complication is bleeding:
  - ◆ 1:10 risk of haematuria
  - ◆ 1:100 risk of a clinically significant bleed
  - ◆ 1:500 risk of endangering the kidney, leading to the need for embolisation and/or kidney removal
  - ◆ 1:1,000 risk of death ...YES, higher than you thought
- There is a 1:20 rate of getting inadequate tissue for diagnosis; even if kidney tissue is obtained, sometimes there is not enough to split into three pieces for all the tests

VITAL POINT

*✳ Most contraindications are relative
but – clotting must be normal*

Aftercare

- Make sure ward staff know the biopsy has happened
- Organise bed rest on back for 12 hours
- Check puncture site
- Monitor vital signs (BP, pulse etc) for haemorrhage, every 15 minutes for one hour, every 30 minutes for two hours, hourly for 4 hours and 2-hourly for a further 12 hours – or according to unit protocol
- Make sure the patient drinks plenty of fluid
- Check for haematuria with a dipstick
- Some units (safely) send patients who've had native biopsies home after 8 hours. This is in low risk patients who are asymptomatic, have normal blood pressure and normal renal function, and have little pain and no visible haematuria post biopsy. Check the patient doesn't live alone
- Make sure the patient has an appointment within 1–3 weeks of the biopsy to review the result. Special stains may take 1–2 weeks to come through

- Ensure the patient has instructions regarding pain and haematuria, and 24-hour contact numbers
- Send a good discharge summary to the referring hospital and the GP

What if . . . the patient bleeds heavily afterwards?

- Tachycardia may be the first sign of bleeding and must be taken seriously
- At a later stage, back pain and shock may occur
- Occasionally heavy haematuria may cause clot colic or urinary retention
- If shock develops, convert the 'group and save' into a 2 (or more) unit crossmatch
- Make sure there is good large bore IV access and ask for help from someone more experienced
- Do an ultrasound scan to see if there is a bleed around the kidney
- If the bleeding continues and is severe or prolonged, angiography is indicated so that the feeding artery may be embolised – inform the surgeon without delay

VITAL POINT

✱ Back pain and/or shock indicate bleeding following biopsy.
Take action! Get help!

And finally

Go to the biopsy meeting to get feedback. Were you right?

Patient education

Ask the patient to explain to you what they understand the procedure will involve. Explain how the biopsy is done, and that only one kidney is biopsied. They need to understand the following points:

- The biopsy will hurt (but 'no more than the dentist'). Local anaesthetic, rather than sedation, is used to minimise this problem

- The two main complications are bleeding (which usually 'settles down') and failure to obtain a big enough tissue sample so the biopsy needs repeating

- You will be in hospital for less than 24 hours if all goes well

- What goes on in one kidney is likely to be happening in the other (not necessarily obvious to all patients)

- A biopsy can cause bleeding, loss of a kidney (meaning dialysis will be necessary) or, in extreme cases, death

- This is a routine procedure in your unit, so staff have had plenty of practice in performing biopsies safely

- You should call the hospital or come back in if you become unwell (particularly if you suffer severe back pain) after going home

- You should avoid heavy lifting, physical exertion and contact sports for one week

- You should not take aspirin or other anti-inflammatory drugs for one week after the biopsy

- If you have not been sent or given an appointment, ask for one

Reference

Boulton-Jones, M (2000) Renal biopsy. In Johnson, RJ & Feehally, J (eds) *Comprehensive Clinical Nephrology.* Harcourt Publishers

3 Renal angiogram

- A renal angiogram involves injecting radiopaque contrast material into the renal blood supply in order to visualise the renal (or renal transplant) artery
- The main goal of contrast enhanced angiography is to confirm a diagnosis of renal artery stenosis and determine its cause
- Intra-arterial injection of contrast medium is the most effective way of investigating renal vascular anatomy
- The procedure carries risks, especially of contrast nephropathy and cholesterol emboli
- There are three successive phases to a normal arteriogram; arterial, parenchymatous and venous. The arterial phase occurs within 2 seconds and the venous phase by 10 seconds

VITAL POINT

* Intra-arterial injection of contrast medium remains the 'gold standard' for investigation of renal vascular anatomy, but risks causing contrast nephropathy

Indications

- Diagnosis of renal artery stenosis, as part of the investigation of renal failure (acute or chronic) or severe hypertension
- Assessment of vascular anatomy of living donor kidney
- Differentiation of a vascular renal cyst from a hypervascular lesion
- Transection of the artery by blunt or penetrating trauma
- Diagnosis of renal vein thrombosis (but there may be easier methods)
- To embolise (and thereby treat or prevent bleeding from) vascular lesions, such as arteriovenous fistulae or false aneurysms (occasionally caused by biopsies)

Before the procedure

Initial tests

Check the patient is 'fit enough' for the procedure:

- It is essential to ensure female patients are not pregnant
- Blood pressure should be less than 140/90 (unless angiogram is being done for high BP)
- Normal INR/APTR
- Order blood tests (baseline FBC – platelet count > 50 is safe – also baseline urea and electrolytes)
- If anticoagulation therapy is required, stop warfarin (4 days before the procedure) and use IV heparin instead. Stop this 6 hours before the procedure
- Assess the possibility of allergy to the dye – ask about previous allergic reactions

VITAL POINT

✻ Renal angiogram is a procedure that carries risk. Make sure that the patient is fit enough to undergo it, and is aware of the risks involved

Preparing the patient

- Explain the procedure, ensuring the patient is aware of the risks
- Ensure written consent has been obtained
- If the patient is not fluid overloaded, some units give 0.9% sodium chloride intravenously at a rate of 1 ml per kg body weight per hour, starting 12 hours before until 12 hours after the procedure
- No solid foods should be taken 6 hours prior to the test. Clear liquids early in the morning of the test are permitted as are necessary medications
- Ask to remove all dental prostheses and valuables, tape wedding ring, remove nail varnish (so you can use oxygen saturation monitor)
- Take baseline and neurological observations, measure foot pulses

- Encourage the patient to pass urine before going to theatre, as dye can cause osmotic diuresis
- Simple pre-medication prior to the procedure – temazepam 20 mg (or appropriate dose) orally

Patient education before the procedure

- A renal angiogram usually takes 1–2 hours. It is performed under local anaesthetic via the femoral artery (in your leg), but if this is blocked the brachial or radial artery (in your arm) can be used
- You will need to lie on your back on an x-ray table
- Your groin will be shaved, and sterilised with antiseptic
- After you have been given a local anaesthetic, a drip needle will be inserted into your femoral artery
- A guidewire is passed through the needle and into the artery. The needle is then removed. A catheter (tube) is passed over the wire
- Both the wire and catheter are placed in correct position using x-ray screening. Dye is injected through the catheter into the artery to the kidney, then the wire is removed

After care

- After catheter removal, apply firm, direct pressure to the puncture site for 10–15 minutes
- Check puncture site
- Monitor vital signs (BP, pulse etc) for haemorrhage, every 15 minutes for one hour, every 30 minutes for two hours, hourly for 4 hours and 2-hourly for a further 12 hours – or according to unit protocol
- Monitor the foot pulses, and compare to other leg
- The patient should lie flat for 6–8 hours, with IV access available following the procedure
- Encourage oral fluid intake, but no solid foods to be taken for 6 hours

Risks

VITAL POINT

❋ Renal function can deteriorate significantly after the procedure, particularly if the patient develops contrast nephropathy

Contrast nephropathy

- This is the most important short term risk of angiography, as it can worsen renal function

- Incidence of worsening renal failure varies from around 2% in people with no known risk factors and 5% in those with mild renal failure, up to 50% in people with severe renal failure and diabetes

- Typically, contrast nephropathy starts within 24 hours of the procedure, peaks at day 3–5 and returns to baseline within 2 weeks

- The development of contrast nephropathy increases hospital mortality particularly in those who do not regain baseline function

- There are no trials comparing prehydration versus no prehydration, although this has now been accepted as standard practice

- There is no role for the addition of any other agent. Mannitol and/or furosemide increase the incidence of contrast nephropathy and the case for acetylcysteine is still not proven

- Risk factors include: age, male sex, diabetes mellitus, myeloma, dehydration, CRF and a large volume of contrast medium

VITAL POINT

❋ The volume and type of contrast medium used will affect the likelihood and nature of side effects

Cholesterol emboli

- These may be caused by the catheter knocking off an atheromatous plaque from inside an artery. The plaque then breaks up and sends a shower of small cholesterol particles into the kidney, causing acute renal failure (ARF) or acute-on-chronic renal failure (ACRF)

- Cholesterol emboli can be more worrying than contrast nephropathy as the renal failure may be irreversible and the time course more variable
- Other organs are involved in up to 55% of cases resulting in a number of clinical symptoms such as abdominal or muscle pain, nausea and vomiting, gastrointestinal bleeding and angina
- Cutaneous manifestations include purple toes, livedo reticularis, petechiae or necrotic areas of ulceration
- Serum abnormalities (eg raised ESR/CRP, raised amylase, leucocytosis, hypocomplementaemia, elevated liver enzymes and eosinophilia) may alert you to the diagnosis
- The time course is more variable than for contrast nephropathy, with a rapid decline in renal function seen in one third of patients and a more slowly progressive course seen in the remainder

Haematoma

- Occurs in about 25% of patients, around the arterial puncture site
- Can lead to pain or swelling in the groin

Other risks

- Allergic (potentially fatal) reaction to the contrast medium
- Dissection of the renal artery, causing partial or complete occlusion

A recent review of angiography found a 25% occurrence of haematoma and pain at the puncture site. There were no recorded deaths. With balloon angioplasty to the renal artery, the risk of death was 0.5%. Reaction to contrast medium occurred in 2% of patients.

Contraindications

- Previous reaction to radio-contrast media
- Uncorrected bleeding disorders
- Pregnancy

Alternatives to renal angiogram

- Renovascular disease is the cause of ESRF in 6.9% of patients across the age range, but of 11.9% in the 65+ age group
- It is difficult to diagnose, and renal angiogram is still the best technique despite its risks
- However, a renal angiogram should only be carried out if a definitive diagnosis is essential or if it will lead to treatment

Other radiological techniques

- Doppler ultrasound
- Magnetic resonance angiogram (MRA)
- Spiral CT or CT angiogram

None of these techniques are totally reliable. So, apart from a renal angiogram, clinical suspicion is probably the best alternative.

Factors strongly indicative of atherosclerotic renovascular disease

- History of smoking
- Evidence of atheroma elsewhere in the body
- Low level proteinuria
- Asymmetric kidneys shown on ultrasound
- Renal/femoral bruits
- No other obvious cause of renal failure
- Hypertension that is difficult to control
- Deterioration of renal function after initiation of ACE inhibitor/AII blocker treatment, particularly when the patient is dehydrated

VITAL POINT

If it is essential to make a definitive diagnosis, a renal angiogram will need to be ordered. This also allows for intervention

Patient education

Ask the patient to explain to you what they understand the procedure will involve, then tell them the following:

- There are risks associated with this procedure, mainly from possible bleeding (which in rare cases can be very severe) and bad reactions to the dye injected into the bloodstream

- There is a small but significant risk that the procedure will cause your kidney function to deteriorate faster than expected, or even lead to your early death. If your kidney function is made worse, you may need dialysis earlier than expected

- However, this is a routine procedure in your unit, so staff have had plenty of practice in performing renal angiograms safely

- The procedure is usually performed in the x-ray department. It takes 1-2 hours and will not involve a general anaesthetic

- Local anaesthetic will be used, resulting in numbness. You will need to lie flat for 6-8 hours after having the angiogram done

- Don't eat anything solid for at least six hours before your angiogram, and wait until the doctor or nurse says you may eat again afterwards

- You will be able to go home the next day if all goes well

- Take it easy after the procedure. You shouldn't drive for at least 24 hours, or lift anything heavy for three days

- Call the hospital if you feel faint, have a lot of pain or a swelling in your groin, or develop strange rashes on your feet

References

Greco BA, Breyer JB (1997) Atherosclerotic ischaemic renal disease. *American Journal of Kidney Disease*, 29:167-87

Murphy SW, Barrett BJ, Parfrey BS (2000) Contrast nephropathy. *Journal of the American Society of Nephrology*, 11:177-182

4 Assessment of acute renal failure

- Acute renal failure (ARF) is a sudden deterioration (occurring over days or weeks) in kidney function. There is no universally accepted definition
- Patients with chronic renal failure can get superimposed ARF (acute-on-chronic renal failure or ACRF)
- Acute tubular necrosis (ATN) is the most common cause of ARF you are likely to see
- The majority of patients have had major surgery, major bleeding and major sepsis
- Approximately 5% of hospital admissions have a raised creatinine level
- ARF is usually transient and most patients regain baseline kidney function. In ATN, renal function usually starts to recover after 10–14 days
- ARF accounts for 10% of patients entering long-term dialysis programmes
- Glomerulonephritis and systemic vasculitis may be among the most interesting causes of ARF; they are not the most common
- 50% die – yes, a lot!

VITAL POINT

✱ Outside of a renal unit, refer a patient with ARF immediately

Causes

- ARF can be classifed into three groups:
- Pre-renal – this is caused by ineffective perfusion of kidneys which are otherwise structurally normal, eg:
  - ◆ Hypovolaemia

- ◆ Cardiac pump failure
- ◆ Other causes of hypotension
- ■ Renal – results from structural damage to the glomeruli and renal tubules, eg:
  - ◆ ATN (the most common causative condition)
  - ◆ Glomerulonephritis/vasculitis
  - ◆ Tubulointerstitial nephritis
- ■ Post-renal – obstruction of the urinary tract anywhere from the calyces to the urethral meatus, eg:
  - ◆ Prostatic hypertrophy/carcinoma
  - ◆ Bladder tumour/gynaecological malignancy
  - ◆ Neuropathic bladder

Specific causes

- ■ The most common causes of ARF seen in hospital are:
  - ◆ Pre-renal failure
  - ◆ Acute tubular necrosis (ATN)
  - ◆ Obstruction

VITAL POINT

* The 'Surgical Triad' – post-operative volume depletion, infection and nephrotoxic drugs – is a common cause of hospital-acquired ARF

- ■ Elderly people are particularly vulnerable to obstruction, myeloma and renovascular disease
- ■ Glomerulonephritis and vasculitis can affect all age groups
- ■ Glomerulonephritis may present as the nephritic syndrome. This comprises haematuria, proteinuria, hypertension, oedema, oliguria and uraemia

Sometimes ESRF presents acutely. When this happens, psychological care of the patient is critical.

Assessment of ARF

The two most important aspects of management are the recognition and treatment of life-threatening complications. These are:

- Hyperkalaemia
- Pulmonary oedema

The management of these conditions is discussed in the next chapter.

History taking

The history is very important (probably more important than the examination). Ask about:

- Prescribed and non-prescribed DRUGS. Drugs are responsible, at least in part for up to 30% of all hospital-acquired cases of ARF. Certain drugs are particular culprits, eg ACE inhibitors and AII blockers (vasoactive effect), penicillins (interstitial nephritis), gentamicin (tubular toxicity), NSAIDs (vasoactive effect, tubulointerstitial nephritis, papillary necrosis)
- Ask the patient whether they are taking any over-the-counter or herbal medicines too
- Recent angiogram (any type) or IVP (contrast nephropathy from nephrotoxic dye)
- Urinary or gynaecological symptoms (obstruction)
- Family history of renal disease (Alport's syndrome, autosomal dominant polycystic kidney disease)

VITAL POINT

✽ Be sure to establish what prescribed and non-prescribed drugs the patient has been taking recently

It is also important to ask:

- Whether the patient suffers from systemic symptoms such as joint pain, rashes or fever (suggesting vasculitis or connective tissue disease)
- If they have backache or bone pain (myeloma)

The examination

- A thorough clinical examination is also important (even for patients who have been transferred from another ward or hospital)
- Look at the patient – should they be on ITU?
- Do not forget the basics. Pulse, blood pressure, respiratory rate, oxygen saturation and temperature should all be determined within minutes of seeing the patient. It is these observations along with potassium levels (and not fancy tests) that decide the urgency of treatment
- Careful assessment of fluid balance; the two most reliable signs of volume depletion are a low jugular venous pressure and a postural drop in blood pressure
- Look for rashes (vasculitis, cholesterol embolisation)
- Facial appearance (scleroderma, butterfly rash of SLE)
- Heart murmurs (infective endocarditis)
- Pericardial rub (a consequence of uraemia)
- A palpable bladder is an indication of bladder outflow obstruction, and should be followed by a rectal and pelvic examination. Gross macroscopic haematuria usually implies a bladder problem
- Arterial bruits, absent foot pulses or the presence of an abdominal aortic aneurysm make atherosclerotic renovascular disease likely
- Perform fundoscopy (accelerated hypertension)

Some patients are transferred from general wards/hospitals, and may arrive in your unit with a CVP line *in situ*. Use it!

VITAL POINT

✽ Complete anuria is rare and suggests obstruction, vascular catastrophe or (rarely) a severe glomerulonephritis or vasculitis

Tests to organise

Three simple tests, often forgotten, are:

- Urine dipstick
    - The presence of blood and proteinuria is highly suggestive of glomerulonephritis or vasculitis
    - Their absence almost excludes it – you need to know this *now*
- Urine microscopy
    - Red cell casts are diagnostic of glomerulonephritis
- ESR/CRP
    - If raised, this implies infection or an underlying systemic disorder such as vasculitis
    - An ESR > 100 suggests myeloma

The following tests (the acute screen) should be carried out:

- Haematology
    - Full blood count and film (haemolytic uraemic syndrome/ thrombotic thrombocytopenic purpura). It is important the film is examined by an experienced observer, particularly if the platelet count is < 100
    - ESR
    - Clotting
    - Hb electrophoresis (sickle cell screen) in Black patients

VITAL POINT

✱ An inappropriately low, or rapidly falling, Hb suggests myeloma, HUS/TTP or bleeding

- Biochemistry
  - Profile – you need to know the potassium level *now*
  - CRP
  - Glucose (diabetes mellitus)
  - Serum immunoglobulins (IgA nephropathy) and electrophoresis (myeloma)
  - Creatinine kinase (rhadomyolysis)
  - Blood gases if the patient is unwell (metabolic acidosis)
  - Urine for Bence-Jones proteinuria
- Immunology
  - ANA and dsDNA (SLE)
  - Complement factors C3 and C4 (SLE, infective endocarditis, cryoglobulinaemia)
  - Anti-neutrophil cytoplasmic antibodies (Wegener's granulomatosus or microscopic polyangiitis)
  - Anti-glomerular basement membrane antibodies (Goodpasture's disease)
- Microbiology/virology
  - Blood cultures (infective endocarditis)
  - Hepatitis B/C (urgent, not usually for diagnostic reasons, but to protect other patients, nurses, yourself and your colleagues)
  - Antistreptolysin-O titre (post-streptococcal glomerulonephritis)

If glomerulonephritis/vasculitis is a high probability, phone the laboratory and ask for the ANCA, antiGBM and ANA/dsDNA to be done urgently (ie, you need a result *today*)

- Imaging
  - ECG (hyperkalaemia, recent myocardial infarction)
  - Chest x-ray (pulmonary oedema, pulmonary haemorrhage and/or infection)
  - Renal ultrasound (obstruction) – within *12 hours* of admission

VITAL POINT

*✱ You must know the results of three tests within a short
time of the patient being admitted: 1. Urinalysis
(within minutes); 2. Potassium (within 1 hour);
3. Renal ultrasound (within 12 hours)*

Patient education

- Acute renal failure is rare but treatable

- If they ask . . . 50% die (25% if on a renal ward, the 50% figure includes
  ITU patients with ARF). You can tell the patient this (and should if
  they ask). But you may need to qualify it, by explaining (if this is true)
  that *their* type of ARF has a better outlook, and why

- It is normal to be confused and unable to think straight – this will
  improve

- Recovery can take place in 10–14 days, but it can take weeks or even
  months; 2–4 weeks in hospital is normal

- Most patients will regain the full function of their kidneys

- Sometimes the kidneys do not recover and permanent treatment will
  be needed; this will mean regular dialysis and the possibility of a
  kidney transplant in the future

Reference

Glynne, PA & Lightstone, L (2001) Acute renal failure. *Clin Med JRCPL*,
1: 266–73

5 Management of acute renal failure

- You should always begin by asking yourself three questions:
  - ◆ Are there life-threatening complications (hyperkalaemia or pulmonary oedema, intravascular volume depletion)?
  - ◆ Does the patient need dialysis and/or admission to ITU?
  - ◆ What is the pathology?
- Make sure all ward staff know the patient has ARF
- Order daily blood tests
- Ring your specialist registrar or consultant

VITAL POINT

✳ Contact the acute haemodialysis nurse as soon as you know you have a patient with ARF coming in, if there is any possibility they will need dialysis

Life-threatening complications

Hyperkalaemia

- Hyperkalaemia can cause death due to cardiac dysrhythmias (especially ventricular tachycardia and fibrillation) – therefore the patient should be attached to a monitor
- The risk of hyperkalaemic cardiac arrest can be assessed by the ECG
- As the serum potassium rises, the following occur:
  - ◆ Tenting of T waves
  - ◆ Reduced P wave with widening of QRS complex
  - ◆ Disappearance of P wave
  - ◆ Sine wave pattern (pre-cardiac arrest)

Treatment of hyperkalaemia is required when the serum potassium is above 6.5 mmol/l, or at a level of 6–6.5 mmol/l with ECG changes (any change more severe than tenting of T waves). Immediate treatment comprises:

- 10 ml 10% calcium gluconate IV over 60 seconds and repeated until the ECG improves (this acts to stabilise the myocardium)
- If a central line is in place, give by that route. Otherwise, give through large bore peripheral access so as to avoid delay
- Nebulised salbutamol 5 mg
- 50 ml 50% glucose and 10 units of soluble insulin IV over 10 minutes (to drive the potassium into the cells)
  - ◆ May be repeated 2 hourly as necessary
  - ◆ Blood sugars (BMs) should be monitored hourly
- 50–100 ml 8.4% sodium bicarbonate IV over 30 minutes (also drives the potassium into the cells)

These are temporary measures only. If hyperkalaemia does not improve rapidly then renal replacement therapy (haemodialysis/haemofiltration) will be required.

VITAL POINT

✱ Test potassium level and order an ECG as soon as you see a patient with ARF

Pulmonary oedema

This is the most serious complication of salt and water overload in ARF. Initial management is no different to pulmonary oedema in patients without renal failure.

- Sit the patient up and give high concentration oxygen
- Then give furosemide 80 mg IV, followed by 250 mg IV if no response
- Morphine 2.5 mg IV
- It is extremely important to reassure the patient; panic will make the situation worse

Unless a diuresis can be induced, haemodialysis or haemofiltration will be required.

Intravascular volume depletion

- Maintenance of fluid volume homeostasis is essential in the management of ARF

- The two most reliable signs of volume depletion are a low jugular venous pressure and a postural drop in blood pressure. If you are in any doubt, monitor the CVP with a central line

- Individualised prescriptions for fluid are necessary. The fluid infused should mimic the nature of the fluid lost

VITAL POINT

** Continuous clinical assessment is necessary
to ensure correction of volume depletion
and avoid volume overload*

- Once the patient is euvolaemic, intravenous normal saline should be given at a rate equal to the fluid output (eg urine, diarrhoea) plus 30 ml/hour to account for insensible losses

- Daily weighing helps to assess the fluid balance

Does the patient need dialysis?

- Urgent renal replacement therapy is required if the patient has:
  - Hyperkalaemia greater than 6.5 mmol/l or 6-6.5 mmol/l with ECG changes
  - Pulmonary oedema unresponsive to medical management
  - Metabolic acidosis causing circulatory compromise
  - Uraemic encephalopathy, pericarditis or bleeding
- There is no absolute level of urea or creatinine at which you dialyse

*** *The only two absolute indications for dialysis
are* hyperkalaemia *and* pulmonary oedema**

What is the best way?

- Conventional intermittent haemodialysis may be suitable for the patient however patients who are haemodynamically unstable may require continuous renal replacement therapy, usually carried out in the ITU

- The patient now needs a haemodialysis catheter. You must consult an experienced renal physician at this time

  - Think about where the catheter should go

  - Use a femoral line initially if APTR/INR > 1.5 or platelets < 50

  - At night, especially if the person putting it in is tired, it is safer to put in a femoral line – particularly if the patient is very breathless and unable to lie flat

Starting haemodialysis

- Patients should start haemodialysis gently (in order to prevent the dialysis disequilibrium syndrome – characterised by headache, confusion, fits and coma)

- 2 hours of haemodialysis on consecutive days, using low extracorporeal blood flows of 200 ml/min, is safe

- You need to ask the nurse to remove (or occasionally give) IV fluids with the dialysis fluid. If the patient is fluid overloaded, no more than 2–3 litres should be removed during the first session

- If the patient has pericarditis, or is bleeding, dialysis should be heparin-free

- Go back and review the patient; this is good practice

- Organise blood tests before finishing dialysis, to check that potassium is in the 'safe range' (below 6.0), and the urea has fallen by 50% at least

- Most patients get more hypoxic 10–15 minutes into the dialysis session if their O_2 saturation level is low – make sure they have oxygen at this time

- Your primary objective is to save the patient's life; but you should also be thinking about the cause of the ARF
- So, do you need to be making provisional plans for a biopsy? (See pages 14-15)
- What problems are easily corrected? (Hypertension, clotting problems, low Hb, platelets etc)

VITAL POINT

** Try to predict the decision to take a biopsy –
make plans for one, just in case*

What if the patient is not getting better?

- Don't panic if recovery is not apparent immediately. The patient is likely to need 2-3 haemodialysis sessions
- Check with the haemodialysis nurse that the dialysis session was technically satisfactory
- The patient should be out of pulmonary oedema, or at least significantly less short of breath after the first dialysis session. If not, then renal replacement therapy should continue in the form of ultrafiltration so that more fluid is removed

Common complications during an episode of ARF

- Pulmonary oedema (again) needing emergency dialysis
- Sepsis commonly as a result of intravascular dialysis catheters and bladder catheters. If the patient is anuric, or knowledge of the urine output is not significantly affecting management, remove the bladder catheter
- Poor nutrition as most ARF patients are catabolic - think about supplemental nutrition early on and link up with the dietitian
- Assess the patient carefully if there are problems, and have a low threshold for seeking senior medical advice

VITAL POINT

A daily review of the charts – looking at vital signs, fluid input/output, weight and the drug prescription – is an essential part of management

Recovery from ARF (especially ATN)

- Oliguria (< 400 ml per day) is common in the early stages
- In the recovery phase GFR remains low while urine output increases (up to several litres in a day, due to reduced tubular reabsorption of filtrate). This is known as the polyuric recovery phase

VITAL POINT

There is no role for dopamine or furosemide as a treatment of oliguric renal failure

Management of the recovery phase

- Examine the patient daily and don't forget to look at the weight chart
- If the patient is unable to keep up with fluid losses enterally, additional IV fluids will be needed; usually equivalent to previous day's urine output, plus 500 ml
- Levels of potassium, calcium, magnesium and phosphate may all fall
- When the recovery is certain, get the dialysis line out as soon as possible to avoid sepsis

Patient education

- ARF is usually reversible
- ARF can last from a few days to a few weeks
- If your kidneys have not regained their function within three months, it is likely they are permanently damaged and long-term treatment will be required
- The symptoms of ARF are fluid retention, nausea and/or vomiting, headache and changes to mental state (such as being more agitated or less responsive than usual), and feeling tired and weak
- Fluid retention occurs because the kidneys are no longer able to balance the body's fluid levels, therefore:
  - A restricted fluid intake may be required
  - Fluid retention can cause swelling in the ankles, feet, hands and around the eyes
  - In severe cases of fluid retention, fluid gathers in the lungs and causes shortness of breath
- Nausea and vomiting are due to the build up of waste in the body (the kidneys normally get rid of excess waste)
- Headache and altered mental state are due to the build up of waste in the body
- Tiredness and weakness are due in part to anaemia, a lack of red blood cells in the body. Red blood cells carry oxygen around the body. Their production is controlled by the kidneys and this will stop if the kidneys are damaged. So you may need a blood transfusion

Reference

Klahr, S & Muller, SB (1998) Acute oliguria. *New England Journal of Medicine,* 38: 671–6

6 Nephrotic syndrome

■ The nephrotic syndrome is a common reason for admission to a renal ward. It presents major hazards to the patient including:

■ Thromboembolic events secondary to loss of haemostasis control proteins (eg antithrombin III and protein S)

■ Increased susceptibility to infection secondary to loss of immunoglobulins

The admitting SHO or nurse will be asked to control symptoms, then find the cause. The 'workup' may eventually lead to a renal biopsy, so think about making plans for that as soon as the patient comes in.

Definition and clinical features

Nephrotic syndrome is defined as:

■ Urinary excretion of 3.5g of protein per day (normal < 150mg/24h)

■ Hypoalbuminaemia – serum albumin of < 30g/L (normal 35–50)

■ Peripheral oedema

VITAL POINT

✱ The definition is arbitrary. Heavy proteinuria (even if not in the nephrotic range) must always be investigated

There may be no symptoms as such, but usually there will be some reason why the patient has gone to seek medical help. Nephrotic syndrome is rarely 'picked up' on routine blood or urine testing, unlike CRF.

Clinical features

■ Those of the underlying cause – eg retinopathy in diabetes mellitus, murmurs in infective endocarditis

- Frothy urine – the onset of this may indicate the onset of the lesion (the protein stabilises the bubbles)
- Muscle wasting – if proteinuria is severe, and of long duration
- Peripheral oedema
- The features of renal disease in general:
  - High BP (but low BP can also occur, raising various possibilities including hypovolaemia, or cardiac amyloid)
  - Rashes in connective tissue diseases
  - Cryoglobulinaemias
- Non specific symptoms – eg malaise

VITAL POINT

It is important to exclude conditions such as cardiac failure and decompensated liver disease, which may mimic nephrotic syndrome

Causes

- Diabetic glomerulosclerosis is the most common cause of nephrotic range proteinuria
- Several primary glomerular diseases account for the great majority of cases in those without diabetes (minimal change glomerulonephropathy, membranous glomerulonephritis, focal segmental glomerulosclerosis). Depending on age, this group accounts for between 60–80% in adults
- Rarer important causes include:
  - Amyloidosis
  - Pre-eclampsia
  - Cancer (mainly associated with minimal change and membranous nephropathy)
  - Systemic diseases (mostly SLE)
  - Drugs (gold, penicillamine, NSAIDs, ACE inhibitors)

* Diabetes mellitus and primary glomerular diseases account for the majority of cases of nephrotic syndrome, but rarer causes should not be overlooked

Complications

- Muscle wasting due to protein malnutrition
- Sodium retention and formation of oedema
- Infections (especially bacterial such as pneumococcal pneumonia)
- Hyperlipidaemia (due to an increase in levels of VLDL, IDL and LDL fractions resulting in elevated serum cholesterol alone or in combination with elevated triglyceride)
- Hypercoaguable state (due to a multitude of factors including low antithrombin III, low factor IX and XI levels, increased platelet reactivity, increased fibrinogen levels and altered endothelial cell function) presenting as arterial and venous thromboses
- CRF, possibly leading to ESRF
- Death – before the modern range of diuretic and anti-hypertensive drugs, patients could (and did) die of nephrotic syndrome, if it was severe

Investigations

- The same battery of tests should be run as for ARF (see list on page 31)
- An under recognised fact is that the APTR is frequently abnormal (prolonged) in nephrotic syndrome. This is not associated with a tendency to bleed – the haemostatic cascade after injury is triggered by the extrinsic system
- Renal biopsy can therefore be safely performed

There are three groups of patients where renal biopsy is not beneficial:

- Young children with highly selective proteinuria
- In long standing type 1 diabetes mellitus with associated retinopathy (the diagnosis will almost always be diabetic glomerulosclerosis)
- In patients on possible causative drugs, which should be stopped

VITAL POINT

* Tests should be carried out as for ARF, but a renal biopsy is unnecessary in certain categories of patient

Treatment

Management of symptoms

- Treatment of oedema:
  - ◆ Treat initially by reducing dietary sodium to 60 mmol per 24 hours
  - ◆ Fluid removal should be controlled and gradual; daily weight is the best measure of progress
  - ◆ Use of diuretics (furosemide) should involve a stepwise approach aiming for weight loss of 1–2 kg /day. Because of the short elimination half life, twice daily dosing is required
  - ◆ If there is no response to furosemide 250 mg twice per day, add a thiazide diuretic (eg metolazone 2.5–5 mg daily)
  - ◆ If there is still no response (poor absorption from mucosal oedema or poor drug delivery from hypoalbuminaemia), use a parenteral loop diuretic. For inpatients, furosemide infusions 5–10 mg/hr can be very effective
- Daily serum potassium with appropriate replacement (eg amiloride 5 mg daily) is important
- Accurate fluid balance measurement
- Reduction of proteinuria (ACE inhibitors or AII blockers are pivotal)
- There is no role for a high protein diet

- NB: Some patients with severe nephrosis are unresponsive to prescribed drugs. Be wary of the possibility of inducing poisoning (and permanently damaging renal function further) by giving excessively high doses of ACE inhibitors or NSAIDs

Specific measures aimed at the underlying cause

- Give prednisolone for minimal change nephropathy

- Hyperlipidaemia can be treated with statins. You don't necessarily have to treat this NOW if you think the disease will go away quite quickly (eg if the patient has minimal change nephropathy and is being treated with prednisolone)

- Management of hyperlipidaemia should follow the same guidelines as for the general population, ie primary prevention of cardiovascular disease. However, there is no direct proof that this policy is beneficial to patients with nephrotic syndrome

- Anticoagulants if serum albumin < 15 g/l. These patients are likely to need warfarin

- If anticoagulation is indicated, use IV heparin if the patient is likely to need a biopsy soon

VITAL POINT

*Treatment measures fall into two categories
– management of symptoms and treatment
aimed at the underlying cause*

What if the patient has diuretic resistant oedema?

- Consult a senior colleague

- Give 20% human albumin 50–100 ml followed by IV bolus of diuretic 1 hour later (this should be tried in those who are hypovolaemic only, for fear of precipitating pulmonary oedema)

- If all else fails, try ultrafiltration

Patient education

■ Normally protein that you eat stays in the blood, and helps make protein in the muscles etc. It is not lost in urine

■ In your condition, that is not true; some of the protein you eat leaks out through the kidney and appears in the urine. So blood levels of protein are low. We don't know precisely why this happens

■ You are likely to have swollen ankles. You will be prescribed diuretics (water tablets) to get rid of the swelling

■ You may also be asked to reduce the amount of fluid you drink

■ A high protein or low protein diet will not help – it has been tried! Try to avoid salt and Losalt, as this will make your medication work better

■ You will also be prescribed tablets to control your blood pressure if it is high

■ You may need a kidney biopsy to tell us which of the many types of nephrotic syndrome you have. This information will help us to give you more specific treatment

■ The outlook is quite good for most cases

Reference

Orth SR, Ritz E (1998) The nephrotic syndrome. *New England Journal of Medicine*, 338: 1202–1211

7 Renal bone disease

- This is also known as renal osteodystrophy and is used to describe the skeletal complications of renal failure
- Renal bone disease occurs in all patients with ESRF and can start early in the course of the disease
- The various types of renal bone disease are osteitis fibrosa, osteomalacia, mixed (osteitis fibrosa and osteomalacia) and adynamic
- Osteitis fibrosa and mixed disease are associated with high bone turnover due to high levels of parathyroid hormone (PTH) whereas osteomalacia and adynamic disease are associated with low bone turnover and low levels of PTH
- Generally, high turnover states are seen in haemodialysis patients and low turnover states in peritoneal dialysis patients
- If untreated or treated poorly, renal bone disease can be debilitating for the patient and give rise to bone pain, skeletal deformity, fractures, pruritis, and metastatic calcification (eg affecting the conjunctiva and causing 'red eye' syndrome)

Pathogenesis

- In CRF, calcium levels fall:
  - partly due to reduced renal phosphate excretion
  - partly because the kidneys fail to activate 25-dihydroxyvitamin D_3 to the more metabolically active 1,25-dihydroxyvitamin D_3
- Hypocalcaemia produced by these mechanisms is a stimulus to the parathyroid gland which respond by producing more PTH
- PTH promotes reabsorption of calcium from bone in an attempt to return the serum calcium level towards normal
- This secondary hyperparathyroidism can ultimately cause the hyperparathyroid glands to become autonomous – this is tertiary hyperparathyroidism
- In addition, 1,25-dihydroxyvitamin D_3 deficiency and hypocalcaemia results in impaired mineralization of bone (osteomalacia)

VITAL POINT

Normal kidney function is necessary for calcium and phosphate homeostasis

Diagnosis

- The 'gold standard' for the diagnosis of renal bone disease is a bone biopsy, but this is mainly a research tool
- Clues to the presence of renal bone disease can come from serum biochemistry (hypocalcaemia and hyperphosphataemia), raised levels of serum intact PTH and circulating alkaline phosphatase
- Alkaline phosphatase is a good marker of osteoblast activity (high values are seen in high turnover states, and low values in low turnover disease)

VITAL POINT

Measuring PTH levels is the best way of diagnosing and monitoring renal bone disease

Treatment

The basic principle of treatment is to get the phosphate down and the calcium up.

Control of serum phosphorus

'Serum phosphate (measured before a dialysis session in haemodialysis patients) should be lower than 1.8 mmol/l'
(Renal Association Standard, 2002)

- A low phosphate diet is a key component, as is adequate dialysis
- If this is insufficient, then prescribe a phosphate binder such as calcium carbonate, or calcium acetate or sevelamer (Renagel)

■ These bind with dietary phosphate, preventing its absorption, and some raise calcium levels. To be effective as phosphate binders they must be taken at mealtimes with food (before, not after)

Control of serum calcium

'Serum calcium, adjusted for albumin concentration, should be between 2.2 and 2.6 mmol/l (in PD patients and pre-dialysis in HD patients)'
(Renal Association Standard, 2002)

■ Serum calcium concentrations need to be maintained at the high end of the normal range in order to suppress PTH
■ If the phosphorus level is in the target range, calcium supplements should be taken between meals or at night

Vitamin D analogues

■ The two types commonly used are calcitriol and alfacalcidol (starting dose 0.25 µg/day)
■ The dose should be titrated to the PTH level
■ The target intact PTH level is 3 to 4 times the upper limit of normal
■ Lower levels of PTH may cause a low turnover state and higher levels a high turnover state
■ The major side effects are hypercalcaemia and hyperphosphataemia

VITAL POINT

✳ Do not give vitamin D analogues in the presence of hypercalcaemia or hyperphosphataemia – extra-skeletal calcification may occur

Parathyroidectomy

Occasionally, medical management fails. A parathyroidectomy may be necessary if the following occur:

■ Hypercalcaemia, despite taking no calcium-containing or provoking drugs, in association with a raised PTH (tertiary hyperparathyroidism)

- Inability to suppress PTH into target range without causing hypercalcaemia (with evidence of bone destruction)

- Calciphylaxis – a serious condition characterised by skin necrosis involving both the trunk and extremities. It carries a very poor prognosis as a result of disseminated infection

- Intractable itching – however, the patient should be warned that a parathyroidectomy may not get rid of this symptom. This is because the pathogenesis of itching is unclear

VITAL POINT

* Parathyroidectomy is a major operation with risks, so is only worth doing if the patient can be expected to live long enough to gain benefit from it

Pre-operative checks

- Check that a parathyroidectomy is indicated

- Some units recommend a vocal cord check

- Pre-operative localisation is likely to be required. Check that the ultrasound/CT/MRI/nuclear medicine scans have been performed, and the surgeon knows the results

- Check whether a high-dose vitamin D analogue (eg alfacalcidol 1–5µg daily) has been prescribed 3–5 days pre-operatively to reduce postoperative hypocalcaemia (not policy in all units)

- It is the surgeon's responsibility to explain the operation to the patient and establish consent

What to tell the patient before the procedure

- Why the operation is necessary

- That the operation will last about 2–3 hours, and a hospital stay of 3–4 days will probably be necessary afterwards

- Check that the patient is aware of the risks of the operation, ie:

  - Temporary or permanent damage to the recurrent laryngeal nerve, causing a hoarse voice (< 1%)

  - There is a 5–10% recurrence of hyperparathyroidism after total parathyroidectomy

- There are different surgical approaches:
  - ◆ Total parathyroidectomy
  - ◆ Near-total parathyroidectomy (removal of 3½ parathyroid glands)
  - ◆ Total parathyroidectomy with auto-transplantation of half a gland in the forearm (now rarely done)

Postoperative management

- Check potassium and calcium levels 2 hours after surgery
- The main post-operative problem is hypocalcaemia ('hungry bone syndrome') which may be severe, rapid (falls within 12 hours of the operation) and dangerous (leading to fitting and/or death), if not spotted and reversed
- Calcium levels should be checked daily for at least 3 days after surgery and weekly thereafter until stable
- When calcium levels fall below the normal range, prescribe calcium supplements and vitamin D analogues. The doses required will depend on the absolute level and rate of fall. Large doses are often needed (eg calcium carbonate 6 g/day and alfacalcidol 1–10 µg/day)
- Intravenous calcium is indicated if the patient develops tetany. This is treated with 10 ml 10% calcium gluconate (into a large vein) followed by 40 ml of 10% gluconate in 1 litre of 5% glucose over 8–12 hours
- In some cases patients need to be discharged on high doses of calcium supplements, and vitamin D analogues. If so, it's very easy to 'overcook' it and make them hypercalcaemic, which can be just as dangerous. Therefore, make sure that patients are discharged with robust arrangements for follow-up of calcium levels
- Arrange for removal of stitches if necessary
- Drains usually come out on a non-dialysis day (if the patient is on haemodialysis)
- Stitch cutters should be close at hand postoperatively

VITAL POINT

✱Hypocalcaemia post parathyroidectomy can be life-threatening – check the calcium level immediately postoperatively, and at least daily thereafter

Patient education

- Renal bone disease is a common complication of ESRF

- It is not usually life-threatening, but the symptoms can be very unpleasant

- In kidney failure, without treatment, the calcium levels tend to be low in the blood, and phosphate high

- Normally, a chemical (called PTH) produced by 4 'parathyroid glands' (in the neck) helps to regulate calcium and phosphate levels. In kidney failure, the blood levels of PTH often go up. If this happens, you have a problem with renal bone disease

- Phosphate binding tablets (eg Calcichew) and vitamin D tablets (eg alfacalcidol) may be prescribed for you, and should be taken as directed. Dialysis can also help to correct the calcium, phosphate and PTH levels

- A transplant usually gets rid of the problem, but it can flare up immediately after the operation, and come back if the transplant ever fails

- If the blood level of PTH is very high, and the calcium and phosphate levels are not coming under control, you may need a parathyroidectomy, an operation to remove the parathyroid glands

- Parathyroidectomy is a major operation that carries risks. Make sure your doctor talks these through with you

- The major postoperative problem is a very low blood calcium level. You will need calcium supplements for life

- When you leave hospital after a parathyroidectomy, make sure your calcium level is measured (and reacted to) within a week

References

Elder G (2002) Pathophysiology and recent advances in the managements of renal osteodystrophy. *JBMR*, 17: 2094-2105

Hruska KA, Teitelbaum SL (1995) Mechanisms of disease: renal osteodystrophy. *New England Journal of Medicine, 333: 166-175*

8 Anaemia and EPO

Why anaemia?

- Anaemia is an almost invariable consequence of ESRF and has a major effect on morbidity and mortality
- Many symptoms experienced by patients with ESRF can be attributed to anaemia rather than uraemia
- In ESRF, anaemia is often multifactorial; the major causes are inappropriately reduced erythropoietin (EPO) levels, haemolysis, blood loss and iron deficiency
- EPO is a hormone that promotes the proliferation and differentiation of erythrocyte precursors in the bone marrow

VITAL POINT

* *Correcting anaemia improves survival and quality of life*

Treatment

- Correction of anaemia is by administration of Recombinant Human Erythropoietin (epoetin or EPO) by injection or – rarely – by blood transfusion
- EPO should be prescribed to predialysis, dialysis and transplant patients when the haemoglobin falls below 10g/dl
- The target haemoglobin should be 11–12g/dl in patients with ESRF. This target is for EPO therapy, and is NOT an indication for blood transfusion
- EPO is given subcutaneously in many patients, as this allows a reduction in dose (compared to the intravenous route)
- It is usually given 1–3 times each week, and may take 3–4 months to reach target levels

- Haemoglobin should be monitored every 1-2 weeks after initiating therapy or after a change in dose
- Once a stable haemoglobin has been reached, monitoring can be done monthly
- To reduce the risk of adverse effects, a haemoglobin increase of 1 g/dl/month is appropriate

'A definition of adequate iron status is a serum ferritin > 100μg/l and < 10% hypochromic red cells (transferrin saturation > 20%)'
(Renal Association Standard, 2002)

- All dialysis patients should receive iron, unless their serum ferritin is greater than 800μg/l, and must remain iron replete - EPO therapy uses up iron stores
- Many patients require regular IV iron therapy, although a small percentage are able to maintain adequate iron stores using only oral iron supplements
- Regular monitoring of iron status (every 3 months) is *essential* during treatment

VITAL POINT

* IV iron therapy must be discontinued for 2 weeks prior to measuring iron status

Resistance to EPO

- Failure to respond to EPO is called 'resistance'
- True resistance is defined as failure to reach target haemoglobin in the presence of adequate iron stores at a dose of 300 units/kg/week subcutaneously
- The main causes of EPO resistance are:
  - Bleeding
  - Iron deficiency
  - Infection
  - Inflammation
- During an episode of infection/inflammation, there is no value in increasing the dose of EPO as this will not overcome the associated EPO hyporesponsiveness

VITAL POINT

** The only common side effect of EPO
is hypertension*

What if the patient suffers from high blood pressure?

- An increase in blood pressure following EPO occurs in approximately 25% of patients
- High blood pressure should be controlled in exactly the same way as for patients who are not on EPO
- It is not necessary to stop EPO therapy on account of hypertension

VITAL POINT

** EPO should only be discontinued in the presence
of hypertensive encephalopathy*

What if a patient comes into hospital without bringing any EPO?

- It is vital that EPO therapy is continued, even during hospital admissions
- Many hospital pharmacies do not stock supplies of EPO, therefore the patient's own supply must be obtained from their home
- As EPO is given intermittently, 1–3 times a week, it should be possible to wait for one day for the supplies to arrive from the patient's home

Patient education

- Anaemia is a common problem for almost all kidney patients

- Anaemia is the term used for a lack for red blood cells in the body

- Red blood cells carry oxygen around the body – oxygen (combined with nutrients from food) provides us with energy

- The main symptoms of anaemia are tiredness, shortness of breath, pale skin, poor appetite, irritability, poor memory and low sex drive (including problems with erections)

- Anaemia is usually treated with 'EPO' injections

- EPO is a synthetic form of the 'hormone' (chemical) that makes the body produce red blood. Natural EPO is made in the kidneys and goes to the bone marrow which it stimulates to make red blood cells

- EPO injections are usually given 1–3 times a week; most patients give EPO injections to themselves

- The most common side effect of EPO is a worsening of high blood pressure. If this happens, you may need to take more blood pressure tablets

- EPO works very well for most people. If it does not work it may be because you have other problems (such as bleeding, infection, or low levels of iron in your body)

- A successful transplant usually makes anaemia better and EPO can be stopped

- Never stop taking your EPO injections, unless your kidney doctor or EPO nurse tells you to

- Always bring your EPO into hospital with you

- Remember to order and pick up supplies in plenty of time, before you run out

Reference

Macdougall, IC (2003) Anaemia of chronic renal failure. *Medicine*, 31 (6): 63–66

9 Peritoneal dialysis and catheter insertion

- Peritoneal dialysis (PD) uses the patient's peritoneal membrane as a semipermeable membrane
- A silastic catheter is inserted into the peritoneal cavity through the anterior abdominal wall
- Inserting a PD catheter is a routine procedure, but one that must be organised properly
- PD catheters can be inserted percutaneously under local anaesthetic or surgically under general anaesthetic. If you were having one put in, which would you prefer?
- The catheter has one or two Dacron cuffs which secures the device and prevents catheter leakage and infection
- PD fluid (dialysate) is infused into the peritoneal cavity under gravity
- Solutes cross from the patient's blood into the dialysate through the peritoneal membrane by diffusion and convection

PD catheter – position inside the body

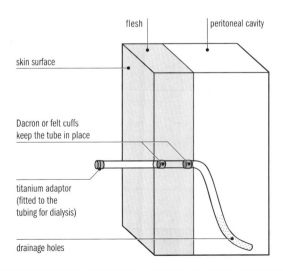

flesh | peritoneal cavity

skin surface

Dacron or felt cuffs
keep the tube in place

titanium adaptor
(fitted to the
tubing for dialysis)

drainage holes

- Excess fluid is removed from the patient by the osmotic pressure within the dialysate
- The usual osmotic agent used in PD fluid is glucose
- After several hours the dialysate fluid is drained out and the process repeated

Who is suitable for a PD catheter?

- Most patients will be suitable. They are unlikely to be suitable, however, if they are very obese, if they have had repeated abdominal operations leading to adhesions, or if they have a history of diverticular disease
- Hernias may need to be repaired
- The patient (or a relative) must be able to perform the dialysis

VITAL POINT

* People with abdominal adhesions or diverticular disease may be unsuitable for PD, as may those who are very overweight

Pre-operative care

- Ensure the patient is capable of performing PD
- Obtain consent
- Prescribe laxatives (senna, lactulose) which should have been started before admission. This helps intraperitoneal catheter placement
- Some units prescribe prophylactic antibiotics (eg vancomycin or cefuroxime). Check your unit protocol
- Ensure that the exit site has been marked (by a PD nurse or doctor) with indelible ink
- The patient should empty their bladder immediately before catheter insertion to avoid bladder perforation

- PD is not usually started until about 10 days after the operation
- Around 25% of PD catheter insertions don't work properly first time, and require another 1-2 operations to sort them out
- It is important to look out for the following warning signs:
  - Traces of faeces in the PD effluent (indicating bowel perforation)
  - Urine draining from the PD catheter (indicating bladder perforation)
  - Excess blood in the PD effluent (some blood is normal, but an excess is indicative of an intraperitoneal bleed)
  - Abdominal pain and fever (peritonitis)
  - Exit site infection
  - Fluid leak around catheter site
  - Postoperative ileus
  - Hospital acquired pneumonia

When are patients sent home or trained?

- This varies from patient to patient, and unit to unit
- Most units send the patient home the day after the operation, and get them to return about 10 days later for training, usually as an outpatient
- Training usually takes a week

VITAL POINT

Check with the PD nurses before sending a patient home. In fact, run most decisions on PD patients past the PD nurses, who may well know more than you

Patient education

- Inserting a PD catheter is a routine procedure, which will be performed by an experienced operator

- It is not suitable for everyone. If you have had several abdominal operations, your peritoneum may be too scarred for effective PD

- If you are very overweight or suffer from diverticular disease, PD may not be suitable for you either

- The procedure involves abdominal surgery and perhaps a general anaesthetic, neither of which are entirely risk-free

- The operation takes less than an hour. If all goes well, you can go home the following day

- You are unlikely to start PD for another 10 days or so

- The wound may hurt initially

- Your bowels may be blocked for a while (referred to as an 'ileus'). You may be prescribed laxatives to keep your bowels regular and prevent problems with poor drainage of PD fluid

- Dressings should be left in place for 10 days unless soiled or wet. They should be changed using strict aseptic technique and preferably by the PD nurses

- It is important to get out of bed as soon as possible after surgery as this lessens the risk of complications (eg deep vein thrombosis, clot on the lung, chest infection)

- There are specific risks – such as bowel and bladder perforation

- Around 25% of patients experience technical problems (such as leaking tubes or poor drainage)

- This means that 25% of patients might need further operations to get it sorted

Reference

Gokal, R & Mallick, NP (1999) Peritoneal dialysis. *Lancet*; 353: 823–828

10 Peritonitis and other problems with PD

- The complications of peritoneal dialysis can be divided into infectious and non-infectious
- The main infectious complications are PD peritonitis and exit site infections
- Non-infectious complications include:
  - Catheter malfunction where there is poor inflow and outflow of dialysate
  - Fluid overload
  - Hernias
  - Fluid leaks around the catheter exit site

Peritonitis

'Peritonitis rates should be < 1 episode/18 patient months'
(Renal Association Standard, 2002)

- The incidence of PD peritonitis has declined over the past decade with the introduction of new technology and improved patient education
- Even so, it remains the main complication of PD
- Peritonitis is one of the main causes of long-term PD failure
- Most patients get about one episode of peritonitis every 18 months. These are usually dealt with by nursing staff on an outpatient basis
- Unlike conventional ('surgical') peritonitis, it is usually a mild illness that does not require a laparotomy
- This is not to say it doesn't require skill to manage – it does

Organisms

PD peritonitis

- The main routes of infection in the peritoneum are from skin contaminants, via exit sites and the bowel
- Skin and exit sites:
  - The most common routes for infection in PD patients
  - Usually introduced at the time of connection or via an infected exit site
  - Gram-positive organisms such as *Staphylococcus aureus* and *Staphylococcus epidermidis* are the most common
  - Staphylococci adhere to the catheter making them difficult to eradicate, thus causing recurrent infection
  - Routine nasal swabbing of patients and staff will help to eliminate the risk of Staphylococcal infections by prescribing mupirocin to those who are positive
- Bowel:
  - Gram-negative infections (from the bowel) – eg *E Coli* – may be introduced as a result of poor hygiene or (transmurally) directly from the bowel
  - The likelihood of this type of peritonitis is greater with increased bowel permeability (eg due to diarrhoea or diverticulitis)
  - Peritonitis associated with diverticulitis often involves more than one organism

Other rarer organisms

- *Pseudomonas* infections occur via skin contamination and are often associated with exit-site infections
- Fungal infection can occur following a prolonged course of antibiotics
- *Mycobacterium tuberculosis*

Surgical peritonitis

- Bowel (or any abdominal viscus) perforation should always be considered if:
  - ◆ Pain is severe
  - ◆ There is a mixed growth of Gram-negative and Gram-positive organisms
  - ◆ The PD fluid is dark or turbid
  - ◆ There is no improvement within 3–4 days

VITAL POINT

＊Severe abdominal pain with dark dialysate implies a perforated abdominal viscus. This is life-threatening – the patient must be seen by a senior surgeon urgently

Clinical presentation

- Often the first sign of peritonitis is cloudy dialysate
- The patient may or may not have abdominal pain and fever
- The exit site and tunnel should also be checked, for signs of infection; and swabs sent if necessary

VITAL POINT

＊Peritonitis often presents with a cloudy bag; the other two classical findings (pain and fever) are not always present

Diagnosis

- Specimens of dialysate are sent for white cell count, Gram stain, and culture and sensitivities
- A white cell count greater than 100/mm^3 (more than 50% of which are polymorphonuclear neutrophils), is considered to be indicative of peritonitis
- An excess of lymphocytes may suggest TB peritonitis
- Eosinophilic peritonitis (an allergic reaction to the dialysate) is present if the Gram stain and cultures are negative and more than 10% of peritoneal leucocytes are eosinophils
- An abdominal x-ray is not helpful, as gas under the diaphragm may occur in PD patients whether or not they have peritonitis

Treatment

- Empirical ('best guess') therapy is started in all patients with a cloudy bag before cultures are back, due to the time taken for laboratories to grow organisms
- Treatment should cover both Gram-positive and Gram-negative organisms
- There is huge variation in treatment protocols, from unit to unit. Get to know yours
- PD peritonitis is usually treated by intraperitoneal (IP) antibiotics, injected into the PD fluid before it is instilled into the patient. Some protocols also use oral drugs
- Units will have different treatment protocols. However, some current examples of initial treatment regimes include:
  - Vancomycin or cefazolin IP (this covers Gram-positive organisms), *and either:*
  - Gentamicin IP, *or* ciprofloxacin PO, *or* ceftazidime IP (these cover Gram-negative organisms)
- The exchange containing the antibiotics should be left to dwell for 6 hours
- Depending on the organism the length of treatment is between 10 and 21 days

- When the organism has been identified, one antibiotic can often be stopped
- Gentamicin levels should be measured on day 2, then every 2 days (and the drug not given if > 2 mg/l). You are trying to treat the organism without risking ototoxicity
- Fungal, pseudomonas and TB peritonitis need catheter removal; and antimicrobial therapy (eg fluconazole and flucytosine for fungal peritonitis; or gentamicin for pseudomonas; or conventional TB therapy)
- Antibiotics should not be given for eosinophilic peritonitis

VITAL POINT

✳ 10–30% of cases are culture negative but still require 10–21 days of antibiotic treatment

What if the patient's condition does not improve?

- Patients should start to feel better and clearing of the PD fluid should start within 48 hours. If there is no improvement within 3-4 days, then:
  - ◆ Fluid should be retested for white cell count, Gram stain and culture
  - ◆ Check antibiotic sensitivities
  - ◆ Consider an unusual organism such as a fungus, pseudomonas or TB
  - ◆ Is this surgical peritonitis?

VITAL POINT

✳ For fungal, pseudomonas and TB peritonitis, or if the patient is very unwell, take the catheter out. If the patient is not getting better after 7 days, take the catheter out, whatever the organism

Other infective complications

Exit-site infections

- These may present with a purulent drainage – with or without erythema of the skin – at the exit site of the PD catheter

- A culture of the purulent discharge should be obtained to identify the causative organism. The most common organisms are *Staphylococcus aureus* and *Pseudomonas* species

- Antibiotic therapy (flucloxacillin 500 mg, 4 times/day PO) may be started if the infection looks severe, however it may be delayed until the results of the culture are available. Gram-negative organisms are treated with ciprofloxacin 500 mg twice/day PO

- Erythema alone does not require treatment

- Treatment should be for a minimum of 2 weeks

'Tunnel infection'

- Usually, but not always, this presents as an extension of an exit site infection into the catheter tunnel

- Swelling, pain and redness over the subcutaneous tunnel may be observed

- Diagnosis can be confirmed by ultrasound where fluid is seen collecting around the catheter

- Treatment is similar to that for exit-site infections

- Tunnel infections do not often respond well to antibiotic therapy; it is usually necessary to remove the catheter (especially if there is peritonitis)

PD catheter malfunction

- If in doubt, call the PD nurse

- A 2-litre bag of dialysate should take approximately 15 minutes to run into the peritoneal cavity and approximately 20 minutes to drain out

- Kinks in the tubing are the most common cause of poor draining and rectification is simple

- Fibrin formation is another common cause of a blocked catheter. Fibrin can often be removed by 'milking' the tubing. Heparin (5000 units/litre) should be added to the dialysate for the next few cycles as a preventative measure
- If this fails, an abdominal x-ray should be performed. This will show the position of the catheter and whether any significant faecal loading of the bowel is present
- If the catheter is in the pelvis and there is no faecal loading, urokinase (25,000 units in 10 ml sodium chloride 0.9%) can be infused into the catheter lumen (under aseptic conditions) and left for 2–4 hours
- If constipation is present, stimulant laxatives such as sodium picosulphate should be prescribed (stimulant laxatives help treat constipation, non-stimulant laxatives help prevent recurrence)
- Constipation is a major cause of poor drainage, particularly in new PD patients
- Catheter migration towards the diaphragm is also more likely with constipation, and can cause poor drainage
- If the catheter is in a poor position due to constipation, this is usually rectified once the constipation is resolved. It can also be due to the omentum becoming attached to the catheter tip. An omental attachment makes the catheter migrate out of the pelvic cavity, which is difficult to resolve without surgical intervention

VITAL POINT

✳ Help your patient to avoid constipation.
Encourage a high fibre diet, regular exercise
and non-stimulant laxatives

- In the event of any potential or actual contamination, leak or other issues, if in doubt:
  - ◆ Drain the fluid out of the patient
  - ◆ Clamp and cap the line with appropriate products
  - ◆ Speak to the PD nurse as soon as possible

Patient education

- The most common complication of PD is infection. If you think you are developing an infection either around your catheter site or internally, *contact your PD nurse without delay.* Don't wait for the next day or Monday morning

- Keeping your PD catheter and the exit site clean is very important. Be scrupulous about hygiene and following your PD nurse's advice

- Dark or cloudy dialysis fluid is a serious sign. Contact your PD nurse immediately if you see this

- A little blood in the dialysis fluid is not a problem if you are a woman having your period. But blood for no obvious reason should be reported

- Another problem with PD is poor drainage. Tell your PD nurse if your exchanges are taking longer than usual or if your catheter appears to be obstructed in any way

Reference

Keane WF, Bailie ER *et al.* (2000) Adult peritoneal dialysis related peritonitis treatment recommendations: 2000 Update. *Peritoneal Dialysis International*, 20: 396–411

11 Vascular access for haemodialysis

The maintenance of good, durable vascular access for haemodialysis is essential for well-being and survival. If vascular access cannot be achieved the patient will eventually die. There are three types of permanent vascular access:

- Primary arteriovenous fistula
- Polytetrafluoroethylene (PTFE) grafts
- Dual lumen cuffed (tunnelled) catheters

The primary arteriovenous fistula is the most effective form of long-term vascular access.

Arteriovenous fistula

A fistula

1 Normal vein

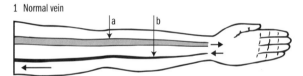

a Artery takes blood to the arm and hand
b Vein takes blood from the hand and arm

2 Vein diversion

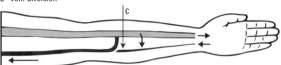

c A diversion of the vein is formed, linking it to the artery in the forearm

3 Vein thickens

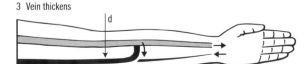

d The vein thickens beyond the link, and can now be used as a fistula

- A fistula is established by connecting an artery to a nearby vein by direct surgical anastomosis

- It is created either at the wrist or at the antecubital fossa, using the radial artery or brachial artery respectively

- Although both the artery and the vein may retain their normal connections, the new opening between the two will cause some arterial blood to shunt into the vein because of the pressure difference

- This causes thickening of the fistula vein wall ('arterialisation') and enlargement of the lumen

VITAL POINT

* Avoid venupuncture or cannulation at the wrist or forearm veins in any renal patient. They may be needed later to make a fistula

Creating a fistula: why and when?

'At least 80% of prevalent HD patients should be dialysed using a native arteriovenous fistula'
(Renal Association Standard 2002)

- Arteriovenous fistulae are preferred because of their relative longevity (60–90% are functioning at 3 years) and lower susceptibility to infection when compared to PTFE grafts and dual lumen tunnelled catheters

- Good fistulae can tolerate high flow rates, leading to efficient dialysis, which in turn leads to improved health

- Availability of a suitable vein remains the limiting factor in up to 30% of patients, meaning another form of vascular access is required

- Preparations for vascular access should be made when the creatinine clearance has fallen to 25 ml/min or within a year of anticipated dialysis. Arteriovenous fistulae need at least 6–8 weeks to mature before the fistula is ready for use and ideally be left for 3–4 months

- In the UK there are two reasons for creating them 'early':
  - They have a significant failure rate, so you need time to have 'two goes' or more
  - Most units don't have enough access surgery time. There is often a three month waiting list for routine access surgery, so you need to get your patient in 'when you can'

Radial or brachial?

- While arteriovenous fistulae are the access of choice, someone (usually a consultant) will have made the decision as to whether a radial or brachial fistula is best for a particular patient

Carrying out the procedure

- Fistulae are usually created by a surgeon, though some physicians still do them
- They are usually done as day surgery, but occasionally patients require overnight stay
- Anaesthesia may be either local or general
- The procedure takes 1–2 hours
- There are various techniques including a side-to-side, and a side-to-end anastamosis

Clinical assessment

Special investigations

- Most nephrologists now recommend some form of 'vein mapping' with a Doppler ultrasound (or venogram) as part of a fistula workup
- Doppler ultrasound is less accurate than venography for evaluation of central vein structures
- Veins bigger than 3mm wide are more likely to work

Patient fitness

- Even if the procedure is being done under local anaesthetic, it is very important to be sure the patient is fit for surgery by all standard criteria (eg normal blood pressure, no fluid overload):

  - The potassium should not be high (< 6 mmol/l)

  - Aspirin can continue but warfarin should have been stopped and the INR be < 1.5

- See pages 82–83 in the Transplant chapter for more detailed information on ensuring your patient is fit for surgery

- No matter how senior the doctor who has arranged the fistula, don't assume that they have 'got it all right'. The following points in the history should have prompted prior venography because of the high incidence of venous impairment (stenosis, thrombosis):

  - Current or previous subclavian catheter placement of any type in venous drainage of planned access

  - Current or previous transvenous pacemaker in venous drainage of planned access

  - Previous arm, neck or chest trauma or surgery in venous drainage of planned access

  - Multiple previous accesses in an extremity planned as an access site

- In addition there are examination findings (in any planned access site) which should have prompted prior venography:

  - Oedema

  - Collateral veins

  - Differential extremity size

Complimentations

- Thrombosis:
  - Is the most common cause of arteriovenous fistula loss
  - 80-90% are caused by venous stenosis
  - Can also be caused by hypotension, intravascular volume depletion and prolonged compression
  - Rapid surgical intervention can 'save' the fistula

VITAL POINT

* If you think a thrombosis may have happened, call someone senior immediately. Don't leave it until tomorrow – that may be too late for successful intervention

- Stenosis:
  - Is almost always venous
  - Arises as a result of intimal fibromuscular hyperplasia within the first 2-3 cm of the venous anastomosis
- Oedema of the hand and arm:
  - An increase of 2-3 cm in circumference is common, but larger increases indicate venous hypertension due to venous outlet stenosis
- Arterial steal:
  - The limb distal to the fistula is deprived of an adequate blood supply
  - The patient may complain of a cold, weak, numb or painful hand
  - Early recognition is important to preserve limb function
- Aneurysm formation:
  - Aneurysms can be false or true
  - Usually no action is required. But if there is progressive enlargement, or the overlying skin becomes thin, the aneurysmal segment should be excised
- Infection:
  - This is rare. If it occurs, it should be treated with antibiotics for 6 weeks

Other forms of access: grafts

- Grafts are popular in North America
- The workup, from your perspective, is similar
- Their advantage is that they can be used in 2–4 weeks or, if necessary, almost immediately
- Long-term results are not as good as for fistulae

VITAL POINT

* Tell the patient . . . if the buzz stops return to the hospital, immediately, day or night!

- During surgery, your vein and artery (demonstrate) will be connected in order to create a useable entry point for the haemodialysis needles

- The procedure will take around 1-2 hours, and is likely to be done as day surgery using either local or general anaesthetic

- Some pain and swelling is normal. Keep this to a minimum by raising your arm whenever possible on a pillow positioned above your heart for the first 1-2 days

- Your arm may bruise slightly. Do not put heating pads on your arm. Simple painkillers such as paracetamol should help

- When you go home, you can use your arm and hand without endangering the surgery. You can go back to your usual activities such as driving and housework after 2 days, if everything is OK, but take a week off work if it involves anything strenuous

- Don't stop taking your usual prescribed medicines

- There are usually no stitches to be removed. Even so, don't have a bath or shower for a week at least. If your wound gets wet, do not rub it dry, gently pat it with a clean dressing

- A little blood may ooze through the dressing. Don't worry about this unless pus starts coming through as well. If this happens you may have an infection and will need to go back to hospital

- You will feel a buzz (or 'thrill') through the bandage. This is normal, and a good thing – it shows that the fistula is working

- If you stop feeling the buzz, this may mean that the fistula has stopped suddenly, due a blood clot in it. If this happens, you should return to the ward immediately

- Make sure you are not wearing a watch or night garments around your fistula arm. You should sleep on your other side

- Your fistula is your 'lifeline'. Take great care of it!

Reference

NKF-DOQI (1997) Clinical Practice Guidelines for Vascular Access. New York, National Kidney Foundation

12 Complications of haemodialysis catheters

In addition to arteriovenous fistulae and PTFE grafts, vascular access can be achieved using dialysis catheters.

■ Temporary haemodialysis catheters are dual lumen, non-cuffed and non-tunnelled

■ Permanent haemodialysis catheters are dual-lumen, cuffed and tunnelled

■ The cuff, as a consequence of tissue ingrowth, secures the catheter in place and reduces the incidence of infection

■ Temporary catheters are placed when haemodialysis access is required for less than three weeks, or as a bridge to more permanent access

■ Haemodialysis catheters are placed either in the internal jugular vein or femoral vein. They are not placed in the subclavian vein because of the high incidence of venous stenosis that can occur at this site

■ Femoral lines should be at least 19 cm in length in order to reach the inferior vena cava and thus minimise recirculation

VITAL POINT

** Don't use subclavian veins
for any kind of dialysis catheter*

Complications

■ The two main complications of haemodialysis catheters are infection and catheter dysfunction from catheter lumen thrombosis

■ Catheter dysfunction is defined as extracorporeal blood flow of less than 300 ml/minute

Haemodialysis catheter infection

- All catheters carry the risk of bacterial infection
- It is a common and serious problem associated with significant morbidity and mortality
- Infections can involve the exit site, tunnel tract or bloodstream
- The usual organisms are *Staphylococcus aureus* or *Staphylococcus epidermidis*
- Gram-negative organisms can occasionally cause infection, particularly with catheters placed in the femoral vein

Infection of a temporary haemodialysis catheter

- If this is suspected, take blood cultures from a peripheral vein and look for other sources of infection. If no other source is obvious, treat the problem as a catheter infection
- If septic shock is present, the catheter should be removed immediately and antibiotics given (see below). The catheter tip should be sent for culture

VITAL POINT

✳ Remove the temporary haemodialysis catheter and give IV antibiotics if the patient is septic and there is no other obvious cause

- Treat with an empirical antibiotic regime (see pages 78–79). Don't wait for cultures (they may be negative)
- If the sepsis resolves, wait as long as possible (usually about 2 days) before you put in fresh access
- If 'deep-seated' infection is discovered, 6 weeks of appropriate antibiotics may be necessary

VITAL POINT

✳ In patients with persistent fevers or elevated CRP, exclude endocarditis and osteomyelitis/discitis

Infection of a permanent haemodialysis catheter

- This is more complicated than for temporary lines. The first bit is the same, ie take blood cultures from both a peripheral vein and through the dialysis catheter to enable appropriate interpretation of a positive result

- Look for other sources of infection and if no other source is obvious then treat as a catheter infection with an empirical IV antibiotic regime outline (see below). Again, don't wait for cultures

- Catheter exit site infections should be treated with topical antibiotics

What next? Do I take the line out?

- This depends on how important the line is, how many previous episodes of infection there have been, and most importantly, how ill the patient is. If in any doubt, ask a senior

- If the patient is systemically well:
  - Give IV antibiotics and leave the line in
  - Watch closely over the next 24–48 hours. The patient should get better
  - Nonetheless, give 1–2 weeks of antibiotics

- If the patient is unwell:
  - Give IV antibiotics and leave the line in
  - If the patient doesn't improve, or gets worse, the line should be removed
  - Send the tip off
  - Whether the line is removed or not, give 1–2 weeks of antibiotics

VITAL POINT

✱ If the patient is gravely ill, remove the line NOW

Empirical IV antibiotic regime

- This may vary from one unit to another. However, a common regime involves vancomycin 20 mg/kg IV and gentamicin 2 mg/kg IV. One dosing of each may be enough

- Further dosing is necessary when the vancomycin level falls below 10 mg/ml and/or the gentamicin level falls below 2 mg/ml
- If blood cultures are positive, adjust the regime according to the sensitivities of the organism

Haemodialysis catheter thrombosis

- Thrombosis of catheter lumens is the most common cause of haemodialysis catheter dysfunction
- The incidence of catheter thrombosis can be reduced by filling each lumen with heparin 5000 units/ml after each dialysis session
- In some units, the problem of temporary catheter thrombosis is addressed by exchanging the catheter over a guidewire, though this is not a practice of choice everywhere
- Treatment of permanent catheter thrombosis should initially be the administration of intraluminal urokinase. An example of a protocol for urokinase administration is as follows:
  - Attempt to aspirate catheter lumen
  - Steadily inject urokinase (5000 units/ml) into the occluded catheter lumen
  - Fill entire catheter lumen
  - After 30 minutes, aspirate catheter

This will be successful in around 75% of cases. If it is unsuccessful, flow can usually be restored by intra-catheter infusion of urokinase over 6 hours. This should be preceded by catheter imaging with contrast to confirm the presence of thrombus. There should be no contra-indication to systemic urokinase

- If this doesn't work, get someone senior to take the permanent line out

VITAL POINT

❋ Taking tunnelled lines out is as hard, or harder, than putting them in. Get someone senior to teach you

Other causes of catheter dysfunction

These include:

- Mal-positioned catheter
  - This will usually have to be removed
- Fibrin sheath formation enveloping the catheter tip
  - Fibrin sheaths can sometimes be lysed with urokinase infusions or removed by an interventional radiologist using a snare – the patient must be off warfarin
  - As a final measure the catheter can be exchanged over a guidewire (often done with antibiotic prophylaxis)

Patient education

- The two main complications of haemodialysis catheters are infection and blockages
- Catheter infections can be very serious. If you notice reddening, soreness or pus around the tube contact the renal unit straight away
- If your haemodialysis catheter does become infected, you are likely to need treatment in hospital. This is because the cause of the infection needs to be discovered so that the correct antibiotics can be given. The haemodialysis catheter may also need to be removed. You may be in hospital for 1–2 days, or up to 6 weeks, depending on how bad the infection is
- If your haemodialysis catheter becomes blocked, you will not be able to have dialysis as there will be no way of taking blood from your body to the dialysis machine
- You will not know if your catheter is blocked until the nurse attempts to use it for dialysis
- Blockages may be treated by injecting a solution of urokinase into the tube. If this does not work, the catheter will need to be removed and replaced by another one

References

McGee DC, Gould MK (2003) Preventing complications of central venous catheterisation. *New England Journal of Medicine*, 348:1123–1233

13 Transplants

- Renal transplantation is the treatment of choice for many patients with ESRF. It offers a better quality of life (and sometimes a longer life) than dialysis
- The technique involves the anastomosis of a human kidney from a cadaveric or living donor to the iliac vessels of the recipient
- The donor ureter is placed into the recipient's bladder
- Lifelong immunosuppressive treatment is required to prevent graft rejection

A kidney becomes available

- Don't panic – treat it like any other semi-urgent operation
- However it is not just a surgical procedure. It requires the combined skills of a surgeon, transplant co-ordinator, laboratory staff, anaesthetist, theatre staff, physician and nurses. All have to do their job well, for the transplant to work
- You have to put the same amount of effort in every day, not just on the day of the transplant
- If you have to ring the patient, tell them not to eat or drink anything, and to come quickly (without rushing unsafely) to hospital

When the patient arrives

- Place nil by mouth
- Make some calls – call the anaesthetist (request triple lumen central line and remind not to use forearm veins for cannulation), surgeon and tissue typist. Make sure theatres are booked
- Locate the kidney
- Get the patient's notes or call up the database. Read the last few letters

- Make a quick decision regarding dialysis – mainly an issue with haemodialysis patients as PD is a continuous process. Dialysis is required if there is significant fluid overload or the potassium level is high (> 5 mmol/l or according to unit protocol). A 2-hour haemodialysis session may be adequate and is often given heparin-free. If the patient is on PD, ask the nurses to do two exchanges (strong bags) over a 2-hour period. Drain out before theatre

VITAL POINT

✳ *The patient should be euvolaemic at the end of dialysis, as it is easier to operate on full blood vessels and reduces the risk of post-operative thrombosis*

Assessment – clinical

- A thorough general assessment to assess the patient's suitability for transplant should have been performed before they reach the unit
- This will include any history of malignancy or ischaemic heart disease, for example
- While performing an assessment prior to transplant, it is advisable to focus on certain areas that may have changed while the patient has been on the waiting list

History

- What is their normal urine output? Write it down
- Has the patient had any recent infections?
- Are there any potential drug interactions with immunosuppressive drugs (eg azathioprine with allopurinol)?
- Is the patient on warfarin?
- If the patient is on haemodialysis, when was he/she last dialysed?
- What is the patient's ideal dry weight?

*✲ The dry weight is the weight of the patient
in normal fluid balance*

Examination

- Is there evidence of fluid overload?
- How much does the patient weigh? Again, write it down
- Document the peripheral pulses. If they are poor, the pelvic vessels (to which the kidney is attached) may also be poor, so check the surgeon knows
- It is better to 'turn down' an unfit patient than 'waste' a good kidney

Investigations

These will vary slightly from unit to unit. Look at your unit's protocol. They will probably include:

- Full blood count
- Clotting
- Biochemical profile
- Haematology crossmatch (3-6 units)
- Tissue typing crossmatch
- Virology (EBV, CMV, HIV, hepatitis B, hepatitis C)
- ECG and a chest x-ray
- MSU
- Culture
- PD fluid

Tissue typing crossmatch

- Lymphocytoxic antibodies against HLA antigens may be present in the recipient. If these are directed against the HLA antigens of the graft, hyperacute rejection of the graft may occur
- Therefore, analogous to the practice in blood transfusion, a crossmatch of the lymphocytes of the donor with the recipient's serum is performed before transplantation
- If it is positive, it is unlikely that the transplant will be able to proceed

VITAL POINT

If the tissue typing crossmatch is not immediately negative, you must consult a senior

Medication

- This is VERY important. No matter how experienced you are, get a registrar or consultant to check the drug chart BEFORE the patient goes to theatre
- There are two main reasons for medication specific to transplant surgery:
  - ◆ Induction immunosuppression
  - ◆ Prophylaxis

Induction immunosuppression

- All units have different regimes, and there may be different regimes for different types of patient (eg first or second cadaveric transplants, living transplants). Some of the drugs will need to be given before the patient goes for surgery – look at your unit's protocol
- Either way, medication will probably be based around a 'triple regime' of:
  - ◆ Calcineurin inhibitor (ciclosporin or tacrolimus)
  - ◆ Anti-metabolite (azathiprine or mycophenolate mofetil)
  - ◆ Corticosteroid (prednisolone)

Prophylaxis

This will include the prescribing of drugs to prevent:

- *Pneumocystis carinii*
- Cytomegalovirus (if the recipient is CMV negative and donor CMV positive)
- Candida
- Peptic ulcer
- Osteoporosis
- Tuberculosis (in Asian or other 'at risk' patients)

VITAL POINT

✳ Always *get a senior colleague to check the drug chart* before *the patient goes to theatre – no matter how experienced you are*

What to tell the patient before theatre

- First, check with the patient that their consent has been obtained
- Don't frighten them – they will be 'on edge' already
- The procedure will take 2–3 hours
- Demonstrate the site of the operation – the iliac fossa
- Explain they will come back with tubes coming out of the neck (CVP line), the abdomen (wound drain) and bladder (urinary catheter)
- There is usually a stent inside the ureter (though not all surgeons insert one). Explain what a stent is
- They should be able to get out of bed the next day and go home in 2 weeks if all goes well
- If the patient has a PD catheter *in situ*, this will usually be left in to be taken out when the uteric stent is removed (or after 6 weeks), if the graft function is stable
- There is a small risk that the graft won't 'take' and the transplant will not be working after one year; there is also a 30% risk that the transplant will not work at the start, but then 'kick in' later. Some grafts are also lost over subsequent months, but over 90% are still working at one year
- The kidney might be 'rejected' by the body, but rejection can usually be treated successfully

When the patient gets back from theatre

You will need to check the following:

- Full blood count, urea and electrolytes (particularly postassium levels). Repeat 4 hours later. A falling creatinine is the only reliable marker that the kidney is working
- Chest x-ray (for CVP line position and pneumothorax)
- Observations – don't forget the basics:
  - Blood pressure
  - Pulse rate
  - Respiratory rate
  - O_2 saturation
  - CVP
- Urine output
- Wound drains – look for excessive blood loss

What next?

If the urine output is not significantly different from the pre-operative value or starts to tail off, take this seriously. It means there is graft dysfunction. Talk to a senior.

The following possibilities should be considered:

- Hypovolaemia
  - Correct this with colloid initially, using CVP measurements as a guide
- Obstruction
  - Consider blocked urinary catheter
- Transplant artery thrombosis
  - Arrange Doppler studies of the artery immediately

Once the patient is euvolaemic, intravenous normal saline should be given at a rate equal to the urine output plus 50 ml/hr. If the above possibilities have been excluded, then (and only then) label the situation as ATN and consider fluid restriction. Talk to a senior. DON'T wait until the following morning.

** Thrombosis of the transplant renal artery is
heralded by the sudden onset of oliguria*

The long term

Kidney transplants don't last for ever. Depending on the patient's age and
the success (or otherwise) of the current transplant, one or more
additional transplants may be necessary in their lifetime.

Cadaveric transplant, graft survival

- 90% will be working one year after the transplant
- 65% will be working at 5 years
- 35% will be working at 10 years

Living-donor transplant, graft survival

- 95% will be working one year after the transplant
- 75% will be working at 5 years
- 60% will be working at 10 years

Major causes of death for transplant patients

- Coronary artery disease
- Infection
- Malignancy, especially lymphoma

VITAL POINT

** The importance of taking the prescribed immuno-suppressant
medication after a kidney transplant cannot be over-emphasised
to the patient*

Patient education on leaving hospital

- You will need frequent and regular follow up:
  - ◆ Initially, at least 3 times a week
  - ◆ Then reducing to fortnightly by about six months, if the transplant is going well
  - ◆ Eventually (after 2 years) every 3-4 months
- Ring the transplant ward (or the transplant doctor on call) if you are ill or worried, especially if you are vomiting or have diarrhoea, are passing less urine, or have pain in the transplanted kidney
- Take your tablets carefully – it is very important you don't run out
- Don't take any tablets prescribed by doctors other than the transplant team
- Enjoy the freedom your new kidney can give you

Reference

Smith KGC, Willcocks L (2003) Renal transplantation. *Medicine*, 31 (6): 73-77

14 Non-concordance with treatment

- Living with ESRF necessitates a lifetime of concordance with rules and regimens – every hour of every day, every week, month and year
- The restrictions, regimes and rules can be complicated, difficult for patients to understand and hard to remember. Worse still, we keep changing them
- Non-concordance with treatment is a common problem. All patients will at some point fail to take the advice they are given
- About 30% of patients regularly show signs of not complying with treatment guidelines
- It is more common in adolescents and young adults. Other common factors are:
  - Male sex
  - Smoking
  - Less education
  - Single status
  - Depression
  - Low income
  - Lack of social support
  - Co-morbidity

What is non-concordance?

The term can be used to describe a patient who fails to follow the advice of their healthcare professional and is most commonly displayed by patients who regularly:

- Arrive late or fail to attend haemodialysis sessions
- Skip CAPD exchanges or shorten or miss APD sessions
- Contract PD peritonitis due to poor hygiene
- Arrive late or miss clinic appointments

- Are under-dialysed or fluid overloaded
- Fail to take medication as prescribed
- Continue to smoke despite advice to give up
- Do not adhere to a recommended diet

How do I know if a patient is doing it?

- There is no set pattern but blood results, blood pressure and weight gain may reveal under-dialysis and fluid overload, for example
- In transplant patients, the most common form of non-concordance is linked to medication. This can have serious and immediate consequences, resulting in transplant failure

VITAL POINT

Failing to follow advice is difficult for renal patients to disguise

Is it always a 'Bad Thing'?

- Within limits, flouting the rules once in a while can be a good sign. Patients who are obsessed with their disease and treatment may also have problems
- Persistently ignoring advice or failing to comply with treatment regimes can be dangerous or even life-threatening
- In a 10-year study of 64 haemodialysis patients, the behaviour of the patient was directly responsible for 5 (11.6%) of the deaths, by suicide in three cases and non-concordance in two cases

What are the causes?

- Lack of understanding:
  - Patients may either not understand the instructions that they have been given or not understand the implications of failing to follow them
  - The treatment of renal failure is often long term and therefore the consequences of not taking a specific drug or following a particular diet may not be immediately apparent. This can lead to the patient feeling the medication or diet is having no effect
- Long-term effects of fluid overload on the heart are also difficult to appreciate
- Depression:
  - This may be related directly to the treatment or their life in general
  - If life appears generally intolerable, it really doesn't matter to these patients that they take risks
- Defiance:
  - This is often directed towards staff whom they feel are 'nagging'
  - Many adult patients have not been told 'what to do' since they were children
- Denial:
  - This is often a coping strategy for many patients – if they carry on 'as normal' they feel as if nothing has happened

VITAL POINT

Be careful about the language you use. 'Non-compliance' sounds judgemental and may cause further harm

What can you do as a doctor or nurse?

- Recognise and understand the problem. Discuss it with the patient at an appropriate time, preferably at a pre-designated time in a non-threatening environment

- Patients need to recognise and accept the problem before anything can be done. Help the patient do this – endless lectures have no effect and may make the problem worse

- Supply the patient with information (pamphlets, books, website addresses). *Make sure* they *understand* it. Ask questions to gauge understanding and talk to the patients about how they will fit a particular behaviour into their lifestyle. In this way, patients can exert free will, and regain power over their disease

- If you think the patient is depressed, take it seriously and arrange an appropriate referral

- Arrange psychological referral (if you have a good service) for behavioural modification

- Address smoking and weight loss in a non-judgmental way, accepting that constant nagging may have the opposite effect. Would you give up beer or chocolate?

- If the patient has a poor prognosis type of renal disease (diabetes mellitus or renovascular disease) don't be too hard on them. Stopping smoking and losing weight may not have any benefit at this stage in their disease

- Arrange support for young adults, especially if they are isolated

- Carry out research on the causes, effects and possible 'treatments' for non-concordance. Little is known

- Learn to communicate better with patients; go on a communication course if possible; watch good communicators and copy them; learn from poor communicators too

- Remember to take into account the patients' social and cultural background. In particular:
  - Language and understanding
  - Dietary differences
  - Attitudes to illness
  - Family relationships

- If at all possible, it is better to try to prevent the problem in the first place. Give patients choices. Give them some power over their treatment. Give them the knowledge on which to base (educated) decisions

VITAL POINT

✻ Don't assume that, just because you have given out information, the patient necessarily understands it or will be motivated by it

Patient education

- Non-concordance with treatment is common, affecting up to 30% of renal patients

- It can kill you

- You need to learn which things you can safely 'not do', and the situations in which non-concordance is life-threatening

- No one likes being told what to do, kidney patients are no different. However, most people can be persuaded to do something if it is explained to them *why* they must do it

References

Wright, SJ (1998) 'Non-compliance': meaningful construct or destructive, sticky, stigmatizing label? *EDTNA ERCA Journal*, Jan–Mar; 24(1): 35–8

Shulman R, Price JD, Spinelli J (1989) Biopsychosocial aspects of long-term survival on end-stage renal failure therapy. *Psychological Medicine*, Nov; 19(4): 945–54

15 Death and bereavement

- The subjects of death and dying are rarely discussed openly with patients in renal units, although they are vitally important
- Death is a daily occurrence on most renal units
- Up to 20% of dialysis patients die because they choose to stop dialysis. Others choose never to start
- Kidney patients have a much shorter life expectancy than the rest of the population, even if they are being treated. The median survival from the start of dialysis is five years
- People who choose to stop dialysis, or not to start in the first place, should first be fully informed about all possible consequences

VITAL POINT

✱ Patients have the right to as much information as possible in order to make an informed choice

Discontinuing dialysis – the patient's choice

- The subject should be gently explored with the patient. Try to find out if there is anything that can be done to improve their situation
- For some patients, asking to stop dialysis simply expresses a need or problem that could be addressed by counselling or medication
- Referral to a psychiatrist, counsellor or psychologist may help the patient to decide what they really want to do
- Stopping dialysis should not be rushed into, but properly considered
- Some patient's wishes may upset and distress their family – it is important to take their views into consideration too, and allow time for discussion with a religious leader if appropriate
- The final decision to stop dialysis must be the patient's alone. It may be an appropriate decision

What if the patient has a change of mind?

- Patients can change their mind at any stage, and dialysis can be restarted

- It is important to let patients know this is the case when they are making their decision

Patient education before dialysis is stopped

- If you choose to stop dialysis (or not to start it when needed) you will eventually die

- You have every right to make this choice – only you can decide whether your quality of life is sufficient for you to want to go on living

- You should not feel guilty if this is the route you decide to take – choosing to stop dialysis should never be equated with suicide

- The staff at your renal unit will continue to support you in your choice, and do everything they can to make you comfortable

- After stopping dialysis, you may experience symptoms such as nausea, breathlessness and muscle twitching. However, these can be easily controlled with medication

- The last stages of your life should not be difficult or painful. You will find yourself gradually becoming more and more sleepy. One day, you will simply not wake up

Death without choice

- It is harder to plan ahead for many deaths, and on a busy renal unit they can become part of an everyday workload. Don't consider them at best routine, at worst an irritation

- Death management is harder than putting a line in

- When a death has occurred it is easy to think . . . we need to 'get the job done' – ie get body moved, quick decision on the need for a postmortem (PM) examination, quick chat to relatives, inform the GP. Use the bed. Next patient

- STOP what you are doing and THINK. Slow down. As a health professional you have a responsibility to:
  - ◆ Make sure that the quality of a patient's care after death is as high as it was before
  - ◆ Determine what can be learned from the death, especially anything that may be helpful for future patients
  - ◆ Wherever possible, ask yourself the question: 'If I *might* learn something from this death to benefit my next similar patient, why am I *not* pressing for a PM?'

Is it enough to put the death down to renal failure?

- Renal failure is a mode of death not a cause of death, and many patients die of other causes (eg type 1 diabetes mellitus or systemic vasculitis)
- This part of the death certificate has the following components:
  - ◆ Primary cause of death . . . (and duration, but this is not obligatory)
  - ◆ Due to . . . (and duration, but this is not obligatory)
  - ◆ Due to . . . (and duration, but this is not obligatory)
  - ◆ Significant conditions not related to primary cause of death (can be more than one)
- Tick the appropriate box if the death is related to employment. It is important to discuss the implications of this with your seniors as it may influence a widow's pension

VITAL POINT

✱ If you are uncertain about the cause of death, you should refer the case to the coroner

'Hospital' or 'Coroner's' postmortem: what's the difference?

- A Hospital PM is requested of the family by you, in order to gain more information about the patient's death, when the cause is suspected or known. In this case, the SHO usually does the death certificate

- This kind of PM is not a legally required examination to establish the cause of death, which is the purpose of a Coroner's PM

- If the relatives can be traced, their consent must be obtained for even a routine PM, even though this is not technically a legal requirement

- A 'Coroner's PM' is ordered by the coroner, after you have provided information on the case, when a clear cause of death cannot be stated

- Both systems are currently being comprehensively reviewed. Under a new law, consent will be mandatory before organs and tissue are retained for either PM system

Which patients should be discussed with the Coroner?

- The Coroners Rules 1984 and the Coroners Act 1988 govern the duties of Coroners

- This does not mean that all such deaths are thought to be suspicious or sinister. PMs may be ordered if death was sudden or unexpected – for example, the death of a child after surgery or the collapse of an adult for no apparent reason

- The decision to carry out the PM is at the discretion of the Coroner and the Coroner chooses the pathologist. Relatives have no choice over whether the PM goes ahead – it is compulsory to determine the cause of death

- The purpose of the Coroner's PM is limited in law to establishing whether the cause of death was 'natural' or 'unnatural'

- After the PM, the Coroner completes the death certificate

VITAL POINT

* If you think a Coroner's postmortem is necessary, ask for one early in conversation with the Coroner

Guidelines for informing the coroner

A death should be referred to the Coroner if:

- The cause of death is unknown
- The deceased was not seen by the certifying doctor either after death or within the 14 days before death
- The death was violent or unnatural or suspicious
- The death may be due to an accident (whenever it occurred)
- The death may be due to self-neglect or neglect by others
- The death may be due to an industrial disease or related to the deceased's employment
- The death may be due to an abortion
- The death occurred during an operation or before recovery from the effects of an anaesthetic
- The death may be a suicide
- The death occurred during or shortly after detention in police or prison custody

Checklist

- If you are sure of the cause of death, fine. Write the death certificate as soon as possible, and carefully
- If you are not sure of the cause of death, what is your reason for *not* speaking to Coroner?
- If the Coroner has said 'no', what is stopping you from asking the family for permission for a 'hospital PM'?
- Go to the PM if there is one
- Talk to the relatives afterwards. Go in prepared
- Inform the GP at the first opportunity. He/she will not find out otherwise
- Inform the patient's consultant – again, this information needs to be passed on
- Inform the bereavement counsellor or counselling service

VITAL POINT

***If a postmortem occurs, go to it.
It is ignorant to request one then fail to attend**

Telling the relatives

■ You may not be a trained counsellor, but by now you will have done this a few times, and hopefully learnt from your mistakes

■ It is a good idea to have a nurse with you, one who knows the people involved

■ You may be the only person who can really 'put together' the final hours for the relatives, especially if you admitted the patient

■ Always ensure you are able to give relatives privacy when breaking unwelcome news. Think of how they might feel if strangers could see them at such a point

■ The relatives will remember these conversations for the rest of their lives, so think about what you are going to say before you go in. Even make a few notes

■ If you are not sure what to do, or how to say it, ask a senior to do it with you, and go along to learn how (or how not) to do it

Reference

Start RD *et al.* (1993) Clinicians and the coronial system: ability of clinicians to recognise reportable deaths. *British Medical Journal,* 306: 1038–41

Appendix: Hints on prescribing

In the wrong circumstances, life saving drugs can do more harm than good. Checking the drug card in hospital, or the list of drugs in outpatients, is one of the most important things a doctor, nurse or pharmacist can do to help their patient. This appendix makes some dose recommendations for patients in severe renal failure. For the purposes of drug prescribing, severe renal failure is defined as a GFR of less than 10 ml/min.

VITAL POINT

* A good nephrologist IS a good clinical pharmacologist

VITAL POINT

* If you can measure the level of a drug then measure it

Specific drugs

ACE inhibitors/All receptor antagonists
May produce serious hyperkalaemia, and worsening renal failure (particularly with renovascular disease). Check creatinine at baseline, and 2 weeks, after starting the drug, or increasing the dose

Aciclovir
Crystal nephrotoxicty can occur. Give an infusion of saline 1 hour prior to IV therapy. In patients with severe renal failure the IV dose should be reduced by 50%. Oral therapy, in the wrong doses, can make the patient confused or unconscious

Allopurinol

Potentiates azathioprine by inhibiting xanthine oxidase, causing leucopenia, or pancytopenia. Reduce dose by 75% and watch the white count. Avoid the combination if possible. Consider swapping to mycophenolate mofetil. In patients with severe renal failure the maximum dose should be 100 mg daily

Amphotericin

Commonly nephrotoxic when given parenterally. If there is pre-existing renal failure, or if renal failure develops, change to liposomal amphotericin

Antibiotics

The following are commonly prescribed antibiotics with recommendations for dose adjustment in severe renal failure:

Amoxicillin (IV/PO)	Maximum 500 mg 8-hourly
Benzylpenicillin (IV)	25–50% standard dose
Ceftazidime (IV)	Maximum 1g daily
Cefuroxime (IV)	750 mg twice daily
Ciprofloxacin (IV/PO)	50% standard dose
Erythromycin (IV/PO)	Maximum 1.5 g daily
Flucloxacillin (PO)	Maximum 500 mg 6-hourly
Flucloxacillin (IV)	Maximum 1 g 6-hourly
Gentamicin (IV)	1.5 mg/kg loading dose, repeat when level < 2mg/l
Meropenem (IV)	50% standard dose
Vancomycin (IV)	1 g loading dose, repeat when level < 10 mg/l

Aspirin (and all NSAIDs)

Aspirin is generally safe in renal failure, but will increase the bleeding tendency already present in uraemic patients. NSAIDs can cause a reduction in GFR and are best avoided in severe renal failure

Azathioprine

Predominant toxic effect is myelosuppression, but hepatic toxicity is also well recognised. Allopurinol potentiates azathioprine by inhibiting xanthine oxidase, causing leucopenia, or pancytopenia (see allopurinol). Prescribe to be taken at 6 pm in the immediate post-transplant period (to give you time to check today's white count). If white count is less than $4 \times 10^9/l$, or if serial values show a progressive decline reduce the dose or stop the drug. In patients with severe renal failure start with 50% of the standard dose

IMMUNOSUPPRESSION *Don't start or stop this drug, or change the dose, without discussion with a senior nephrologist* **WARNING!**

Beta-blockers

Renally excreted beta-blockers such as atenolol may accumulate and cause bradycardia. Doses should be initially reduced and dose increases based on the heart rate

Calcium channel blockers

Mainly eliminated by hepatic metabolism and are therefore well tolerated

Ciclosporin

Nephrotoxic! Other significant side effects are hypertension, hirsutism and gingival hyperplasia. There are many drug interactions so check all new drugs in *BNF.* Grapefruit or herbal medicines, such as St Johns wort or echinacea, can also increase levels. Check trough level in the morning (ie, prior to morning dose)

IMMUNOSUPPRESSION *Don't start or stop this drug, or change the dose, without discussion with a senior nephrologist* **WARNING!**

Cyclophosphamide

Can cause leucopenia, or pancytopenia. Watch white cell count. In patients over 60 years do not exceed 100 mg daily. If the patient is male and still wishes for children, consider sperm banking

IMMUNOSUPPRESSION *Don't start or stop this drug, or change the dose, without discussion with a senior nephrologist* **WARNING!**

Digoxin

Loading doses are the same. Reduce maintenance dose. It can be as low as 62.5 mcg/day, or even alternate days, in renal failure. Check levels

Furosemide

Use in high dosage if patient has renal failure – doses up to 500 mg/day may be required

Lithium

Lithium has a narrow therapeutic/toxic ratio, so drug levels are very important. Long-term use can lead to chronic interstitial fibrosis and nephrogenic diabetes insipidus. It should be avoided in severe renal failure because of the risk of acute lithium intoxication

Mycophenolate mofetil

Alternative to azathioprine. Bone marrow suppression can occur. Watch the white count and if less than $4 \times 10^9/l$ or serial values show a progressive decline reduce the dose or stop the drug

IMMUNOSUPPRESSION *Don't start or stop this drug, or change the dose, without discussion with a senior nephrologist* **WARNING!**

Opiates

Opiates (including codeine) accumulate in renal as well as hepatic failure. Some are worse than others (eg pethidine). The main problems from accumulation are respiratory depression and drowsiness. In severe renal failure doses should start at 50% of the standard dose

Oral contraceptive

Not contra-indicated in renal failure. Remember predialysis, dialysis and transplant patients can become pregnant

Sirolimus

May be used as an alternative to ciclosporin or tacrolimus, and causes less nephrotoxicity. Its main side effect is hyperlipidaemia. Check levels in the blood

IMMUNOSUPPRESSION *Don't start or stop this drug, or change the dose, without discussion with a senior nephrologist* **WARNING!**

Tacrolimus

Alternative to cyclosporin but still nephrotoxic! Around 30% of patients taking it develop diabetes mellitus, often requiring insulin. Similar side-effects to cyclosporin, but more neurotoxicity and less hypertension and gingival hyperplasia. Tacrolimus can cause hair loss. There are many drug interactions, so check all new drugs in BNF. Check trough level in the morning (ie prior to morning dose)

IMMUNOSUPPRESSION *Don't start or stop this drug, or change the dose, without discussion with a senior nephrologist* **WARNING!**

Glossary of abbreviations

AII blockers angiotensin II receptor antagonists

ACE inhibitors angiotensin converting enzyme inhibitors

ACRF acute-on-chronic renal failure

ADPKD autosomal dominant polycystic kidney disease

ANCA anti-neutrophil cytoplasmic antibody

ANA anti-nuclear antibody

APD automated peritoneal dialysis

APTR activated partial thromboplastin ratio

ARF acute renal failure

ATN acute tubular necrosis

BNF British National Formulary

CAPD continuous ambulatory peritoneal dialysis

CMV cytomegalovirus

CRF chronic renal failure

CRP C reactive protein

CT scan computed tomography scan

CVP central venous pressure

DDAVP desamino-D-arginine vasopressin

dsDNA double stranded deoxyribonucleic acid

EBV Epstein-Barr virus

ECG electrocardiogram

EPO erythropoietin

ESRF end-stage renal failure

ESR erythrocyte sedimentation rate

FBC full blood count

GBM glomerular basement membrane

GFR glomerular filtration rate

HLA human leucocyte antigen

HUS haemolytic uraemic syndrome

INR International Normalised Ratio

IP intraperitoneal

IV intravenous

MRA magnetic resonance angiogram

MSU mid stream urine

NSAID non-steroidal anti-inflammatory drug

OTC over the counter

PD peritoneal dialysis

PM postmortem

PO per oral

PTFE polytetrafluoroethylene

PTH parathyroid hormone

SLE systemic lupus erythematosus

TTP thrombotic thrombocytopenic purpura

Further reading

Cameron JS, *History and Treatment of Renal Failure*, Oxford University Press, 2002

Greenberg A (ed) *Primer of Kidney Diseases*, 3rd ed. Academic Press for NKF, 2001

Johnson RJ, Feehally J (eds) *Comprehensive Clinical Nephrology*. Harcourt Publishers, 2000

Levy J, Morgan J, Brown E, *Oxford Handbook of Dialysis*, Oxford University Press, 2001

Lote CJ, *Renal Pathophysiology*, 4th ed. Kluwer, 2000

McGee H, Bradley C, *Quality of Life Following Renal Failure*, Harwood Academic, 1994

Stein A, Wild J, *Kidney Dialysis and Transplants: the 'at your fingertips' guide*. Class Publishing (London) Ltd, 2002

Stein A, Wild J, *Kidney Failure Explained*, 2nd ed. Class Publishing (London) Ltd, 2002

Thomas N (ed) *Renal Nursing*, 2nd ed. Bailliere Tindall, 2002

Whitworth J, Lawrence JR, *Textbook of Renal Disease*, 2nd ed. Churchill Livingstone, 1988

Renal Association Standards Document,
available on **http://bapn.uwcm.ac.uk/paedtx.htm**

Index

AII blockers 12, 29, 44, 100
acute-on-chronic renal failure (ACRF) 23, 27
acute renal failure (ARF) 14, 23, 43
  assessment 29–30
  causes 27–8
  management of 34–39
acute tubular necrosis (ATN) 27, 28, 39, 86
adhesions, abdominal 58
albumin 41, 45, 49
alfacalcidol 49, 50, 51, 52
alkaline phosphatase 48
allergic reactions 21, 24, 64
Alport's syndrome 29
amyloid 16, 42
anaemia 7, 10, 40, 53–4, 56
anastamosis 71
aneurysm 20, 30, 73
angiogram 20–26, 29
antibiotics 58, 63, 64, 65, 66, 73, 77, 78, 80, 101
anticoagulants 21, 45
antithrombin III 41, 43
arterial steal 73
arteriovenous fistula 20, 69–75
  brachial 69, 71
  radial 69, 71
aspirin 15, 19, 72, 101
atheroma 23, 25
autosomal dominant polycystic kidney disease (ADPKD) 9, 11, 29
azathioprine 102

Bence-Jones proteinuria 32
beta-blockers 102
bicarbonate 35
biochemistry profile 32, 83

bladder 28, 30, 38, 58, 59, 60, 81, 85
bleeding 15, 17, 18, 19, 20, 24, 26, 27, 31, 36, 37, 54, 56, 101
blood pressure 7, 12, 13, 16, 17, 21, 30, 36, 46, 55, 56, 72, 84, 90
bone biopsy 48
bowel, perforation 59
breath, shortness of 10, 40, 56
bruits 25, 30
'buzz' 74, 75

calcichew 52
calcitriol 49
calcium 39, 47, 49, 51, 52
calcium carbonate 48, 51
calcium channel blockers 102
calcium gluconate 35, 51
candida 84
cannulation 70, 81
cardiovascular disease 12, 45
catheter 22, 23, 66–7, 69–70, 72, 80, 85
  malfunction 61, 66–7, 76
  permanent 76, 78
  temporary 76, 77
  removal 66, 77, 80, 98
central venous pressure (CVP)
  line 30, 36, 85, 86
cholesterol emboli 20, 23–4, 30
chronic renal failure (CRF) 7–13, 41, 43, 47
ciclosporin 84, 102
clotting 15, 17, 31, 38, 83
Cockcroft-Gault equation 8–9

communication 92
complement factors 32
connective tissue disease 29, 42
consent 16, 21, 50, 58, 85, 97
constipation 67
contrast nephropathy 20, 22, 23, 24, 26, 29
coronary artery disease 87
Coroner 96–9
  informing 98
creatinine clearance 8, 70
creatinine level 27, 86
crossmatch
  haematology 83
  tissue typing 83, 84
CRP 24, 31, 77
cryoglobulinaemia 32, 42
cytomegalovirus (CMV) 83, 84

Dacron cuffs 57
death
  cause of 96, 98
  certificate 97, 98
deep vein thrombosis 60
dehydration 23
depression 91, 92, 103
desamino-D-arginine vasopressin (DDAVP) 15
diabetes 8, 11, 12, 13, 23, 32, 41, 42, 43, 44, 92, 96, 103, 104
dialysate 57, 58, 61, 63, 64, 66, 67
dialysis, choosing to stop 94–5
discitis 77
diverticular disease 58, 60, 62

Vital Diabetes
Third Edition   £14.99
Dr Charles Fox and Mary MacKinnon
This handy reference guide gives you all the backup you need for best practice in diabetes care, and includes all the vital facts and figures about diabetes for your information and regular use, as well as providing patient and carer information sheets that you can photocopy for patients to take away with them.
"Full of the kind of essential and up-to-date information you need to deliver the best practice in diabetes care."
M. Carpenter, Diabetes Grapevine

Providing Diabetes Care in General Practice
Fourth Edition   £24.99
Mary MacKinnon
This practical handbook gives you all the essential information you need to set up and organise health care for people with diabetes in the primary care setting, by allocating tasks to each member of the team. This book also contains clear guidelines for integrating care with the hospital-based services.
"The complete guide for the primary health care team."
Dr Michael Hall, Chairman of Diabetes UK

Kidney Failure Explained
New Second Edition   £14.99
Dr Andy Stein and Janet Wild
This fully updated edition of this complete reference manual gives your patients and their families all the information that they could want about managing kidney conditions, and covers every aspect of living with kidney disease – from diagnosis, drugs and treatment, to diet, recreational pursuits and sexual relationships.
"This book is, without doubt, the best resource currently available for kidney patients and those who care for them."
Val Said, kidney transplant patient

Kidney Dialysis and Transplants – the 'at your fingertips' guide
Dr Andy Stein and Janet Wild   £14.99
This book is a practical handbook for anyone with long-term kidney failure and their families, and answers hundreds of real questions asked by patients with the condition, offering positive, clear and medically accurate advice on every aspect of living with kidney failure.
"An absolute 'must have'"
Timothy Statham, Chief Executive, National Kidney Federation

Priority Order Form

Cut out or photocopy this form and send it (post free in the UK) to:

Class Publishing Priority Service
FREEPOST
London W6 7BR

Please send me urgently
(tick
below)

Post included
price per copy
(UK only)

☐ *Vital Nephrology* (ISBN 1 85959 102 7)   £17.99

☐ *Vital Diabetes* (ISBN 1 85959 088 8)   £17.99

☐ *Providing Diabetes Care in General Practice*
(ISBN 1 85959 048 9)   £27.99

☐ *Kidney Failure Explained* (ISBN 1 85959 070 5)   £17.99

☐ *Kidney Dialysis and Transplants – the 'at your
fingertips' guide* (ISBN 1 85959 046 2)   £17.99

☐ Please send me the new edition of *Vital Nephrology,*
with an invoice, when it is published

EASY WAYS TO PAY

I enclose a cheque payable to Class Publishing for _____

Credit Card: Please debit my   Mastercard ☐   Visa ☐   Amex ☐   Switch ☐

Number _____ *Expiry date* _____

Name _____

My address for delivery is _____

_____

Town _____ *County* _____ *Postcode* _____

Telephone number (in case of query) _____

Credit card billing address if different from above _____

_____

Town _____ *County* _____ *Postcode* _____

*Class Publishing's guarantee: remember that if, for any reason, you are not satisfied with
these books, we will refund all your money, without any questions asked. Prices and VAT
rates may be altered for reasons beyond our control.*

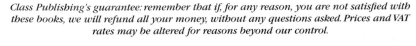

Feedback Form

We, the authors, would welcome your comments on this book.
Would you like more on some subjects and less on others?
Are there additional topics which you would like to see in future editions?
Please help us by marking your comments on this page and sending it to
the publisher, post-free, at **Class Publishing, FREEPOST, London W6 7BR**

Current topics   **More?**   **Less?**

1. *Chronic renal failure (CRF)*   ☐   ☐
2. *Renal biopsy*   ☐   ☐
3. *Renal angiogram*   ☐   ☐
4. *Assessment of acute renal failure*   ☐   ☐
5. *Management of acute renal failure*   ☐   ☐
6. *Nephrotic syndrome*   ☐   ☐
7. *Renal bone disease*   ☐   ☐
8. *Anaemia and EPO*   ☐   ☐
9. *Peritoneal dialysis and catheter insertion*   ☐   ☐
10. *Peritonitis and other problems with PD*   ☐   ☐
11. *Vascular access for haemodialysis*   ☐   ☐
12. *Complications of haemodialysis catheters*   ☐   ☐
13. *Transplants*   ☐   ☐
14. *Non-concordance with treatment*   ☐   ☐
15. *Death and bereavement*   ☐   ☐

Additional topics/Other comments

....

....

....

....

....

May we contact you?

Name: *Occupation:*

Address:

Town: *Postcode:*